THE
FIVE
POINT PLAN

GW00579015

by

James Cooper

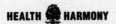

An imprint of

B. Jain Publishers (P) Ltd.
An ISO 9001 : 2000 Certified Company
USA–EUROPE–INDIA

THE FIVE POINT PLAN

First Edition: 2010
1st Impression: 2010

Published by Kuldeep Jain for

HEALTH **HARMONY**

An imprint of

B. JAIN PUBLISHERS (P) LTD.
An ISO 9001 : 2000 Certified Company
1921/10, Chuna Mandi, Paharganj, New Delhi 110 055 (INDIA)
Tel.: +91-11-4567 1000 • *Fax:* +91-11-4567 1010
Email: info@bjain.com • *Website:* **www.bjainbooks.com**

Printed in India by
J.J. Offset Printers

ISBN: 978-81-319-0669-9

Foreword

In the mid 1960's I opened Europe's first health food store at Leicester University and have been spreading the word about organic vegetarian nutrition almost obsessively since then. At the age of 62, I feel more like 42 because I follow a diet and lifestyle that James has encapsulated in his latest book 'The Five Point Plan'. In my opinion, everyone should eat correctly as it is of paramount importance if society is to function properly.

I have started vegetarian societies, campaigned against the globalist health wrecking companies and preached almost daily to the people who visit my shop, many with serious diagnosis. Indeed, we are now treating eminent doctors who have succumbed to cancers and tumours and have failed miserably to cure themselves (Chemotherapy and radiation have a 97% failure rate).

Professionals in the allopathic medical field are coming round to the fact that treating the whole body as opposed to treating specific symptoms is immensely important...a realisation they often seem to come to only after they themselves receive a 'bombshell diagnosis'. You could say my shop (Earth foods in Bournemouth, UK) is something of a 'Patch Adams' institution.

I met James over ten years ago and realised that he was very sincere and hard working in his efforts to help others overcome their illnesses and attain optimum health. In 1997, he saw a photograph of Sathya Sai Baba at the back of my shop and asked about it. I lent him a related book and the very next week he told me with great enthusiasm that Sai had visited him in a dream.

Within three weeks he had flown to Puttarparti, India to see Sai Baba for himself. James's devotion since then seems to have never waned and in my opinion, his work reflects the truth and simplicity of Sai's teachings. For instance, it was James who demonstrated how simply colloidal silver can be made using just three, 9 volt batteries, two silver wires and glass of warm water. I've been spreading that particular gem of information ever since.

James has always studied very hard but never within the confines of a particular course or institution; he is 'autodidactic' in the true sense of the word and has a keen sense of discrimination to 'cut through the rubbish' and synthesise the most important health care information in a way that the average person can understand and utilise.

It's great to see 'The Five Point Plan' in print. It's a book that I'll be recommending to my customers and patients as something that should be studied thoroughly and kept close-to-hand for reference. I was one of the early pioneers of the organic whole food and cellular medicine movement in the 60's and 70's and James is a pioneer, in his own way, of taking natural health care one step further, by making it simple and practical. His desire to serve humanity has resulted in 'The Five Point Plan' and I sincerely hope that it spreads across the world for the betterment of humanity, which I'm sure it will.

Carl Hardman

Foreword

I wish there had been a book available that described the basic needs of the body and how to care for them when the time came for me to start looking for alternative ways of dealing with the health problems that had been afflicting my body since I was a baby. Most babies are born to women who know little or nothing about the nutritional requirements of their bodies or those of their developing babies. My mother did not realize that lack of salt was the condition that caused constant diarrhea and nearly killed me as a baby.

Although she strived to provide nutritional meals to the ten children she had, she ignored the very basic stuff, consumption of adequate amounts of real salt and proper hydration. I wished there had been a book such as 'The Five Point Plan' available then. It would have been priceless to my mother then and to me 20 years ago when I decided to look for alternatives. My friend James has done an excellent job introducing to health conscious people a simple plan to get started on the road to good health and a long, active life.

The five point plan is wisely based on the foundation of good health namely, Water, Salt, Urine, Diet and Exercise. When used properly these elements can be a foolproof guide to monitor and care for the body that can be used by most people who want to live healthy. I specially like the way he simplifies in one phrase the content of my Salt Deficiency book; Chronic Dehydration and Salt Deficiency are the major causes of disease.

I am glad that he introduces the readers to the importance of real salt in the early pages of the book. The World Health Organization knows the importance of consuming adequate amounts of real salt to fight diarrhea and other abdominal conditions that kill millions of babies each year. You often hear press releases describing how

WHO members are distributing salt tablets to fight these ailments in areas where there is no clean water available.

I was born in a third world country but the conditions that led to my being a sickly child are not limited to those of poor countries. Most women in industrialized nations fall into the same category or level of ignorance with respect to the care of babies prenatally and during the first half dozen years of their lives. But this book is not just for mothers with young babies, this volume is also very practical for anyone who wishes to start taking good care of themselves.

Martin Lara
(Author of Uropathy, Salt Deficiency,
The Universal Remedy & Breast Cancer)

Preface

This book reveals the simple practical building blocks of vibrant health, beauty, mental emotional poise, physical healing and longevity in concise layman's language.

The Five Point Plan explores why it is so important to maintain the body's correct water/salt balance, eat the right kind of food, in the right combinations, in the right quantities and also incorporate a sensible exercise regime into a daily lifestyle plan. It outlines the reasons for and methods of utilising ones own urine in accordance with ancient and modern knowledge as well as a system for optimum exercise, both internal and external.

There is so much misinformation and so much illness as a result of false medical practices, yet much of the 'natural health revolution' is also tainted with profit-driven short fallings in terms of effectiveness and accessibility.

Many people overlook the importance of a healthy population. A sick population is not productive and when a society is unproductive it is destined for cataclysm. I see a topsy-turvy world where medical doctors destroy health, lawyers destroy justice, universities destroy knowledge, governments destroy freedom and the major media destroy information. This must stop if we are to ever get out of this mess.

The Five Point Plan details the use of water, salt, urine, diet and exercise in an easy-to-understand and practical way.

I came to my conclusions by experimenting with my own diet and lifestyle, consultations with numerous patients, reading books (both old and new), using the Internet to read lectures/articles and view online educational videos. I have also spent the last eighteen years studying and practising yoga, chi kung and various other health systems.

The message of this book is that illness is primarily the result of unintentional chronic dehydration and incorrect daily habits. With simple modifications of our dietary and lifestyle patterns based on The Five Point Plan we can profoundly transform any society into a truly healthy one; starting with our own personal example.

Acknowledgements

I would like to thank all the tremendous people I have learned from directly and indirectly, whose tireless effort and deep insight are a shining example to us all. In particular I would like to mention Dr. Fereydoon Batmanghelidj for his research into dehydration and salt deficiency, Martin Lara for his crusade in promoting Urine therapy, Swami Sivananda for his beautiful yoga system, life and teachings, Dr. Herbert Shelton for his eloquence and understanding of natural hygiene, Mark Metcalf for his research into and promotion of home-made colloidal silver, Jolyon Sparks for setting me on to the road of health back in the early days, Carl Hardman for kindly sharing his impressive knowledge of nutrition with me and Sri Sathya Sai Baba for his inspiration and guidance.

Publisher's Note

This book reveals the formula by which eveyone can lead a healthy, productive and happy life. Maintaining a correct water/salt balance, eating the right food which is nutritious too, enjoying the benefits of yoga style exercise are among the rules by which everyone can prepare to be healthy, productive and useful to the society of which he is a part. Many people, the author observes, denigrate the value of a healthy population. They overlook the valuable consequences, for society, of a healthy population. The healthy people are not only more efficient at their job, they also are not a burden to their employer or to society. Thus, the employers as well as society can reap dividends.

The book has been written in easy-to-understand language, and not one confined to the Ivory Tower armchair expert. The author knows the pulse of a suffering humanity, and has revolutionized his own personality first. He does not talk down to the reader and is not condescending. He is not dealing with his, but with eternal verities. His argument is careful and methodical. Eschewing junk food and partaking of right and nutritious food will bring victory at the end of a long haul. The anthor has read and researched a great deal before writing this book. The work shall fill, we hope, a long standing gap between the demand and supply curve for good books.

We at B. Jain Publishers fervently hope that the readers appreciate the value of the book and also include in their New Year's good resolutions to try and bring about a change in their lifestlyle, whatever the price, for this makeover in personality will be, when many do it, a decisive factor in India's awakening and renaissance. Many books earlier have proved their influence: Harriet Beecher Stowe's 'Uncle Tom's Cabin' triggered off the American civil war. We at B. Jain in a quiet way pray that 'The Five Point Plan' shows the way ahead to the educated elites.

Kuldeep Jain
C.E.O., B. Jain Publishers (P) Ltd.

Contents

Introduction

Living a life that is free from disease is an accomplishment well worth attaining. Unfortunately, many people today are experiencing a lack of ease in daily living; as we soon notice when we look around at the strained expressions on so many of our faces. The effects of modern day health hazards can accumulate until we forget what it feels like to be completely at ease with our daily life.

The human body is a wondrous creation but it needs to be cared for. All the external wealth and good fortune in the world is meaningless if we are diseased, so the priority must be taken in maintaining our body in good health. This means following the basic practices of personal healthcare and not over-burdening the body with toxic foods and drinks. A burger or fizzy drink may taste nice to some of us but this kind of junk food will lead to disease which will ultimately lead to misery and untimely death. Regular exercise may not seem attractive at first; however the body will not function properly if it is not moved and stretched sufficiently (and it will certainly not thank us for neglecting it). Living in a polluted city may be the best option as far as finding work is concerned, however, it is only a question of time before the pollution and stress brings the body into a state of disharmony and disease. We should all identify those aspects of our lives that are contributing to poor health and start taking the necessary steps. That is what this book is about; identifying the core reasons why there are so many diseases in the world; and finding the simplest, most effective and most universal ways of overcoming these ailments.

In each of us there is a powerful and highly intelligent self-healing instinct that is capable of curing most serious diseases in its own way. Many people with terminal illnesses have been able to successfully support and assist this self-healing instinct and then recover naturally - even from advanced stages of cancer. Through disease we are forced to make changes in our lifestyle, or else we inevitably fall into a downward health spiral, which can cause much unnecessary suffering. Ask most people who have successfully cured themselves by using natural methods and they will tell you that the disease was truly a blessing in disguise. We can all fall into bad habits and if they are not changed, can lead to unhappiness in many different ways, not least physical sickness.

Some people are instinctively drawn to reading books, learning from others and actively being as healthy as they can. They have the 'pull' factor; the idea of radiant health and longevity is appealing to them and drives them forward into living healthily. Other people are not naturally this way inclined, they may have other interests and subsequently do not have the necessary information and motivation to live a healthy life. It is probable (and actually beneficial) that these people encounter some kind of disease, or else the bad lifestyle habits will continue unchecked.

Disease should become the push factor that prompts a general clean up of bad habits and negative attitudes. For instance, let's say Bob is diagnosed with a terminal illness and is given only twelve months to live by his doctor; provided he take the medication. Bob now has a 'push factor' firmly in place. He has two options, either he can blindly believe what he is told, follow the advice and wait to die or he can learn more about the illness and make the necessary lifestyle changes. These changes seemed daunting at first yet he accepted the challenge and didn't give way to despair. In time and with effort he successfully cures himself naturally and in the process, comes to realise many things about himself and the world in general that he probably wouldn't have noticed had the disease not appeared. He firstly learns that we should not always believe what doctors tell us. He also learns that the human body is a phenomenal creation that can heal itself when given a chance. He also learns that once the body has been cleansed, life becomes easier and more joyful. He incidentally learns that a healthy diet is actually much more tasty than living off junk food, that regular exercise is a pleasure and that a clean system and strong immunity means never needing to 'catch a cold' again. All this would have gone unnoticed had it not been for the disease. All this would have been replaced with increasing toxic build-up and ill health had he not needed the prompt to make some changes and get with a healthier plan.

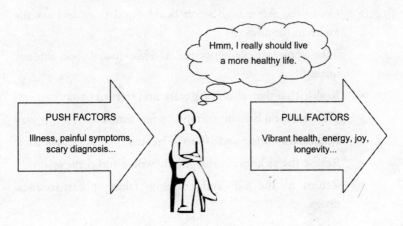

If the human body were a car, disease could be seen as the oil light coming on; don't ignore it. Unscrewing the bulb won't help in the long run either, so avoid medication that suppresses the symptoms without addressing the cause. Disease is our body's way of communicating a message to each of us personally. It is a malfunction warning. It is our issue and our own responsibility to our own body; the vehicle we use to drive through life.

DOWNWARD SPIRALS

Here is a typical pattern of how someone might get sick and hopelessly try to find a 'cure':

> Allow advertising, peer-pressure, cultural norms etc to influence diet and lifestyle habits.

> Gradually get sick.

> See the local medical doctor and take the prescribed drugs.

> Slowly, start to realise that the drugs are actually making the condition worse and/or creating new problems in the body.

> (Repeat last few steps a few times).

> Go to the major high street health food store and ask the assistant for advice.

> Take some supplements for a while (usually of inferior quality).

> Realise that they also don't work and start to panic.

> Visit the local holistic therapist a few times.

> Feel better during and after the treatments but not for long.

> Realise the sickness is still getting worse and panic again.

> Return to the GP and continue taking pharmaceutical drugs.

- Give up hope of ever attaining health.
- Die slowly, painfully and prematurely having never learnt the health lesson.

So, if we add up the personal, financial and emotional cost of being increasingly sick for years; possibly for decades on end the figure is extremely high.

- Days off work
- Paying for prescriptions
- Paying for dietary supplements
- Paying for holistic therapy
- Increasing sense of disempowerment
- Daily physical pain
- Interrupted sleep
- Depression

If only this person had realised that his main problem was that:

- He was not getting any proper exercise.
- He was trying to quench thirst with coffee and sodas.
- He was eating cooked, denatured and chemicalised food.

PRE-REQUISITES FOR HEALING

This book deals with key holistic approaches to disease and would not be complete without the mention of our correct attitude and how important it is as a pre-requisite to healing. Our physical health reflects our various attitudes to life; attitudes we may not consciously be aware of.

For instance, an attitude of 'life isn't particularly important' will promote poor lifestyle habits such as convenience eating. Disease comes along and we are forced to re-evaluate how important we feel our life is. For many people a serious disease is an important catalyst for a change in personal attitudes towards life. These people changed their attitudes and in turn changed their lifestyle habits, which in turn lead to a physical healing and rejuvenation. It may not be easy to change deeply ingrained habits and face physical suffering from such a philosophical standpoint (especially if you have been diagnosed with 'terminal' disease) however the truth remains that our attitudes must change if we are to heal ourselves effectively.

We often have a deep-seated fear of changing our attitudes, which is understandable. Breaking bad habits by changing the way we view life is stepping into the great unknown; who knows where it will lead? To the person who has eaten junk food and drunk alcohol every day for the last twenty years, a diet of vegetarian whole foods and herbal tea may well seem very unattractive. Food and drink is an emotional crutch to many of us and overcoming lower dietary tendencies (such as overeating whenever we feel depressed or drinking when we feel stressed) does not come easily. It is not the process of stopping the junk food or alcohol that is the hard part; we can simply stop buying it. The hard part is changing our attitude sufficiently for us to actually step out into action and stick with our decision even during emotionally difficult periods. Taking time to intuitively think about our life and the situations we create for ourselves is important. Knowledge is also important because changing our attitudes is much easier when we understand more about what a human being really is and how healthcare really works. What you don't know can hurt you and never more so than in today's modern world.

Those who have successfully changed bad attitudes to life will often say that making the necessary changes was 'easy, I just decided one day to change'. Once the attitude or belief system is 're-programmed', then the challenge of creating health and rejuvenation in our lives can be joyous and successful. Notice the people who harbour negative attitudes and compare them with people who are more positive; which ones seem healthier and happier?

VERY BRIEFLY...

> Attitude is important because...

Unless it is positive we will never realise our potential to live healthily and happily. It is part of the cure or wish to be cured.

> Water is important because...

We are primarily made up of water. Our brain is said to be up to 86% water. When the body is dehydrated it gives signals which are generally known as 'diseases'. When dehydrated, the body will compensate by squeezing the colon to extract the moisture from the impacted faecal matter that is stored there. This water is then pumped all around the body causing blockages in the lymphatic system and ultimately leads to disease and suffering; this is just one of the many ways the body desperately tries to retain water, even if painful symptoms are the result.

> Real salt is important because...

It contains dozens of life-giving minerals and is an integral part of our blood. Without it water cannot get into the cells of the body. This results in unintentional chronic dehydration and its many related complications.

> A healthy diet is important because...

You are what you eat. Hippocrates said: 'Food shall be your medicine and your medicine shall be your food.' Staying healthy is impossible when degraded; chemically altered and/or cooked foods are taken into the system regularly.

> Fasting is important because...

It gives the body the time and internal conditions needed to rid it of the accumulated toxins and rebuild health.

> Urine is important because…

It contains the exact information that our body needs to stimulate itself back to health. The urine contains over one thousand beneficial ingredients, is mentioned more times than any other substance in the Hippocratic texts and far from being a waste product; it is actually a highly purified and sterile form of blood. It is the ultimate 'bio-feedback auto-stimulator'.

> Regular exercise is important because…

A primarily sedentary lifestyle is damaging to health and well-being. Internal exercise (such as chi kung) develops the bio-electro-magnetic energy (chi/prana) which forms the invisible basis for physical life. External exercise (such as yoga postures) oxygenate and invigorate the whole body whilst toning the muscles and loosening the joints.

ATTITUDES TO HEALING COMPARISON CHART

Chart 1.1

Negative attitudes	Positive equivalent attitudes
I always get sick.	I get sick sometimes but I am working on it.
Why do I always have to get sick? It's not fair.	Why do I always get sick? I must find out.
Who cares about health? I might get run over by a bus tomorrow.	I really must get healthy, I'll probably live longer and be happier if I do.
You never know what information to believe about healthcare.	I'll learn about the various approaches and see which ones feel right to me.

I'm too old to change my ways.	I must change my ways as I don't have the excuse of ignorance any more.
We all have our cross to bear.	Life can be easier if I change my attitudes towards it.
No one is perfect.	We are all capable of relative perfection.
I can't afford to live healthily.	Healthy living is not about spending money; it's about changing attitudes and making simple lifestyle changes.
It's not fair, I do not deserve to be sick.	This health challenge is providing me with the perfect opportunity to learn important lessons about myself.
Healthy living is boring.	Healthy living is mark of true happiness and maturity.
Healthy food tastes bad.	Enjoying junk food is a sign that I have deviated from what is natural and in my best interests.
I can't see myself sticking to a healthy program.	I will start to change the way I see myself and foolishly impose imaginary limitations on my capabilities.
I'm too busy to bother with it all.	I'm too busy so things will have to change; starting with my attitude.
It's always the most enjoyable things in life that are unhealthy.	Health debilitating habits are not the pinnacle of human enjoyment – there must be more to life.

A pill for every ill.	For every disease in society there is a solution in nature.
What you don't know can't hurt you.	Knowledge is power; over myself and over the hidden dangers of modern life.

AS YOU THINK, SO YOU ARE...

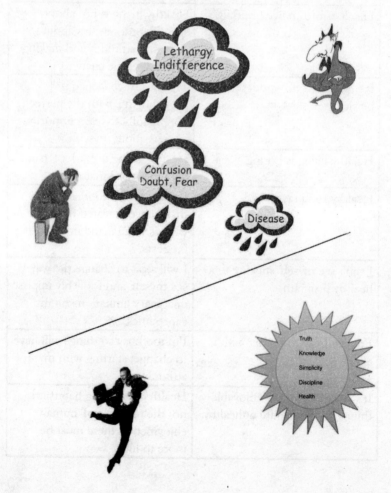

THE WISDOM OF OUR ELDERS

'It is more important to know what sort of person has a disease than to know what sort of disease a person has.'

- Hippocrates

Throughout history, healers and teachers have given health and lifestyle advice to anyone who wished to listen. Examples come from Buddha, who said:

'Disease has no energy save what it borrows from the life force of the organism.'

Or in other words, we are directly responsible for the diseases that affect us personally. We can't carry on leading toxic lifestyles, blindly following the status quo, harbouring negative thoughts and expect to get away with it. Modern medicine looks for external culprits to blame disease on yet Buddha said quite the opposite in a variety of different ways.

Many of us are aware of the stories of Jesus and his miraculous healings yet how many take the time to consider his prophetic words:

'All that I do, you too will do...only much more.'

I suspect he was talking about each and every one of us and the potential we all have to heal ourselves and others – if we only cared enough to realise it.

Louis Pasteur said:

'Le germne n'est rien, c'est le terrain qui est tout.'

(The germ is nothing, it is the soil/terrain that is everything)

This is reflected in Albert Schweizer's remark :

'Serious disease doesn't bother me for long; I am too inhospitable a host.'

A clean, well-nourished, well looked-after, well-hydrated body has a strong immune system and does not fall victim to illness nearly as readily as a weakened system would.

The overall health of the population is in a shocking state which is why 'disease' is so widespread. I believe it is time we all focussed on developing immunity from now on. This means getting properly hydrated with pure water, quitting toxic habits and replacing them with wholesome foods and lifestyle choices.

Lao Tze, in the Tao Te Jing said:

'A great healer heals with the minimum of medicines. The superior healer knows how to heal the first, even without any medicine.'

Many people who are actively involved in healthcare know very well the mind's ability to both create and cure disease. It has been said that:

'It is part if the cure to wish to be cured.'

A combination of good advice on the part of the healer and a strong will to get better on the part of the patient has been a powerful success formula since time immemorial.

THE HUMAN BEING

The human body is a truly amazing creation, which heals itself when given the chance to do so. Why bombard this amazing body with all manner of medications, herbs, supplements and therapies to try to make it function in a particular manner? These approaches invariably lead to future complications, as they do not account for the fact that the human body is naturally self-healing.

In order to help understand what a human is, we need to look at the Sanskrit roots of the word 'human'.

'Hu' refers to 'God', 'object of worship'.

'Manava' means a few different things. One is 'not new' or 'ancient' (Ma=not, Nava=new). Another meaning is 'one who lives without ignorance' (Ma=ignorance, Na=without, Va=lives). According to the authority of the Vedas, this is because the Divine Principle (the Lord, God) exists within mankind.

Therefore, we can see that the word 'Hu-man' refers to a divine being.

So following the true meaning of the word human, does it not follow that our body is capable of healing itself without unnecessary interference? Perhaps this is an over simplistic view point but even if it is, the fact remains that simple solutions to problems are always desirable over complicated ones.

'It is a wonder how the different organs of the body discharge their different functions. The heart performs its functions with utmost regularity and rhythm. It pumps the blood at the right time in the right direction. The lungs and digestive system in the body perform their functions perfectly. In this marvellous creation of God, the functioning of the body is the most wondrous.'

'Most illnesses can be cured by simple living, simple exercise and by intelligent control of the tongue.'

- Sathya Sai Baba

THE SIMPLE TRUTH ABOUT WHAT NEEDS TO BE DONE

An overview of the simple healing approach described in this book can be summarised in three points:

> ➤ Stop the diet and lifestyle habits that lead to the health problem in the first place.

> ➤ Provide suitable internal and external conditions to facilitate the body's self-healing mechanisms.

> ➤ Be disciplined and patient, having faith in the body's self-healing mechanisms.

In many cases of disease, the body needs to be left alone. Often a liquid elixir or food-state supplement can be useful (such as colloidal silver or spirulina) and in most cases, urine is a most universal health booster.

> ➤ Stop the diet and lifestyle habits that lead to the health problem in the first place.

After learning the basics of natural health and healing, identify those foods, drinks and habits that are damaging to health and eliminate/reduce them step by step. Be vigilant and rigorously honest with yourself during your diet/lifestyle self-analysis.

> ➤ Provide suitable internal and external conditions to facilitate the body's self-healing mechanisms.

Keep the body well hydrated by working out your own particular optimum water/salt levels. Eat primarily raw/lightly steamed whole foods, salads, sprouts etc and provide deep rest for the body by fasting and relaxing properly. Re-introduce your own urine by drinking, dropping under the tongue and/or massaging into the skin.

> ➤ Be disciplined and patient, having faith in the body's self-healing mechanisms.

It is a real test of discipline to control our diet and lifestyle, yet the results are worth the effort manifold. Knowing this will make the task of cultivating the necessary discipline to attain health and vitality easier. Patience wins eventually, so don't be impatient for a cure if you have a chronic health complaint or wish to lose weight etc. In reality, the system outlined in this book often leads to rapid healing however some conditions take more time to cure. In times of weakness, sit quietly, smile inwardly and rest assured that the body is an effective self-healing entity.

THE HEALING RESPONSE

Also known as the healing crisis, the healing response can be defined as:

'An intense temporary condition, which occurs before healing as accumulated toxins are released from the body.'

When the body makes the change over from a toxic lifestyle to a healthy one, there may well be some noticeable 'side-effects' that occur, particularly within the first few months. This is nothing to be too concerned about as it is simply the result of all those accumulated toxins being released from the cells and tissues and being expelled by the immune system.

This can lead to a wide range of symptoms, as detailed in the chart below.

Chart 1.2

Head	Dullness, headache, pain
Face	Eczema, fluid retention, swelling, pain, skin rashes, tenderness
Eye	Itchiness, congestion, watering
Ear	Itchiness, swelling, earache, excessive wax build-up, discharge, sinusitis
Nose	Mucus, pus, stuffiness, bleeding, temporary decrease in sensitivity, swelling

Mouth	Bad breath, dry lips, swollen lips, eczema around the lips
Teeth	Gum bleeding, gum swelling, toothache
Tongue	Tenderness, swelling, eczema, green/yellow coating, inability to taste properly
Throat	Sore, phlegm discharge, cough, pain, itchiness, swelling, thirst, fever, hoarseness
Chest	Pressure, pain, symptoms of cold
Oesophagus	Nausea, vomiting, feeling of choking
Stomach	Pain, feeling of fullness, nausea
Intestines	Pain, feeling of fullness, gas, constipation, diarrhoea, dark or sticky stool
Anus	Bleeding, pain, haemorrhoids
Skin	Itchiness, pimples, eczema, eruptions, boils, sores, fluid retention, swelling, internal bleedings, dead skin, perspiration, unpleasant smelling sweat
Whole body	Fatigue, general discomfort, listlessness, drowsiness, insomnia, melancholy, irritability, stiff shoulders, lumbago, inflammation of joints, tenderness, dull pain in any part of the body, local numbness/spasm, muscle pain, lymph gland swelling or pain, general pain/swelling.

Providing that enough water is being drunk throughout the change over into a healthy diet and provided that complete fasting is not undertaken recklessly, the healing response should not be too painful. Drinking urine also helps to ease the symptoms of the healing response.

HOW THE FIVE POINT PLAN DEVELOPED

Early on in life I had developed a keen interest in natural healthcare, spending much of my spare time researching, experimenting with and practicing various forms of healing. I spoke with healers and health advisors from many different schools of thought and listened carefully to what they said and how they said it. I also took a mental note of their personal health, facial expressions etc.

After about fifteen years of enquiry, I became acutely aware that financial profit was clouding the discernment and integrity of many professionals. I also became aware that the truth behind real health is far more simple (and far less profitable) than most of us realise. The Five Point Plan is my offering to anyone who genuinely wants to get healthier and overcome disease.

Realising that most people are suffering from same kind of illness, I felt that an easy to remember, easy to understand and concise system of natural healthcare would be a useful tool to incorporate into my healing endeavours. The central London based holistic health centre in which I worked was an excellent place to develop such a model. Patients would come from all over the UK for health food, advice and therapies; many of whom were literally 'at the end of the road'.

I saw cancer patients who had been given months to live by their GP, AIDS patients who's immunity was so compromised that their teeth were falling out, multiple sclerosis patients who were losing control of their motor responses and chronic arthritis patients who could barely get three hours sleep each night due to the excruciating pain that had become part of their life.

With the work of Dr. Batmanghelidj firmly in my mind, I would always ask the questions 'how much pure water do you drink each day?' and 'what sort of salt do you have in your diet?' before any others.

Invariably, the patient either had an aversion to drinking water, or was not aware of the difference between table salt and real salt, or was on a salt-restricted/salt-free diet or a combination to all three.

I said to Tony at the centre, 'Do you realise that just about all these people who come .to see us are chronically dehydrated?' He agreed with me, and added, 'They're eating rubbish as well.'

I ran it over in my mind and said... 'water'.. 'salt'.. 'diet', then Tony added 'If they get into urine therapy more, their lives would change so quickly.' I agreed, 'Yes, and just a little yoga, or gentle stretching, or whatever, even for just a few minutes each day would speed the process up as well.'

The system was taking shape! 'Right!' I said, 'I'm going to make a set of simple leaflets that outlines the basic things that patients can do, without the need for a series of consultations, to get started with changing their state of health.' The Five Point Plan emerged and I'm still promoting it today.

➢ Water

➢ Salt

➢ Urine

➢ Diet

➢ Exercise

This is an excellent starting point for anyone to learn how to take care of his or her health. A basic understanding of the five principles can also make anyone capable of helping others to get healthier.

We had over three thousand diet/lifestyle books in our bookshelves and I had chosen many of them myself, but how could I expect our patients to read with the same enthusiasm that I and other members of staff did? For many patients, a quick flick through the tabloid newspapers was the only reading they had done for years. My first step was to make a single page information sheet that gave a very brief overview of the five areas, with recommended reading and related websites.

This is how the introductory leaflet looked:

The 5 Point Plan

An Overview

The 5 Point Plan is based on 5 core areas of health and healing, namely Water, Salt, Urine, Diet and Exercise.

Through study, conversations, observations and work with patients, we have come to the following conclusions:

Unintentional chronic dehydration and salt deficiency are the major causes of disease.

Natural and raw whole food keeps the body in good health and can lead to dramatic healing. Abstaining from food for certain periods of time (fasting) is a way to speed up healing and detoxification of the body.

Correct exercise and exposure to fresh air and sunlight are key factors for health and healing.

Urine therapy (or 'Shivambu' or 'Amaroli') is possibly the most advanced and powerful health system in recorded history.

The modern medical system - from the local GP to the international drug companies to the World Health Organisation (WHO) - is controlled by a 'medical mafia' of corrupted and powerful individuals.

The health hazards of modern day living are both lethal (in the long-term) and un-noticed by the majority of the population.

The appalling health of the general population reflects a mental, emotional and spiritual degradation of society.

The vast majority of disease in the world can be cured cheaply, harmlessly and easily by following the guidelines of the 5 Point Plan.

The sheet provided patients with a starting point and gave them a much better chance of recovery, even if they were unwilling to receive therapy, consultations or read books about health. I had also made easily copied information sheets about water, salt, diet, urine therapy, exercise and health hazards, which were freely available to any patients who were interested.

In only ten or fifteen minutes, the basics of the plan could be conveyed to a patient and leave them feeling like they'd received valuable advice, which I was sure they had.

'The five point plan is a very good one. I like it as an introduction to a path to health. Many people need to be educated with respect to the basics needed to promote and sustain good health.'

- Martin Lara, author of Uropathy, Salt Deficiency, The Universal Remedy and Breast Cancer.

The following are transcripts of typical conversations between a patient and me during a set of brief Five Point Plan consultations:

FIRST CONVERSATION: WATER & SALT
(Five minutes)

Me: Hi, how are you?

Patient: Not so good.

Me: What's the problem?

Patient: My joints hurt a lot, I've had rheumatoid arthritis for a long time and I don't have any energy these days.

Me: OK, how much pure water do you drink each day - not tea, coffee, cola - just water?

Patient: Oh, um, well I guess I have 2 or 3 glasses.

Me: And tea or coffee?

Patient: Definitely, I like to drink tea in the day.

Me: How many cups?

Patient: About 5 or 6.

Me: And how many sugars in each cup?

Patient: 2.

Me: Hmmm, that's a lot of tea and sugar. That's about 10-12 teaspoons of sugar each day in your tea alone. Did you know tea was a diuretic drink?

Patient: No.

Me: Yes, you pee out more than you drink in so it doesn't really quench your thirst; it actually makes you more dehydrated.

(At this point I noticed a change in the patient's facial expression)

Patient: Oh right, I didn't know that.

Me: No, most people don't. 2 or 3 glasses of water each day is not nearly enough, you are totally, chronically dehydrated! I'll tell you more about that later. What kind of salt do you have in your diet?

Patient: Well, the usual sort, the one from the supermarket.

Me: You mean the one that you can pour out easily through a shaker?

Patient: Yes.

Me: That's not salt; it's sodium chloride plus a few dodgy chemicals. It tastes a bit like salt but it's not salt.

Patient: Well, I don't put much on my food anyway.

Me: That's not the point, the point is that by denying your body the real salt each day, you are missing out on up to 85 essential elements such as silver, selenium, gold etc.

Patient: So which salt do I need to get?

Me: You need to get REAL salt, un-refined, un-processed salt. It can either be rock or sea salt, but it must be natural. You can get it from decent health food shops, supermarkets etc.

Patient: How much should I take?

Me: Approximately a third of a level teaspoon per litre of water you drink. That's the small spoon, not the big one. Also, remember it's a third of a level teaspoon, not a heaped one.

Patient: So, do I have to put the salt in my water?

Me: You don't have to, but it's a good idea to have some salt water each day as this has special health benefits, which brings me back to how much water you are drinking - you really must drink more!

Patient: How much? I don't really like drinking water by itself.

Me: You're sick, your body will not work properly if you don't drink enough water, so it's not really about your personal tastes, and it's about what you need to do to get better. What is your body weight?

Patient: About 11 stone.

Me: The general formula is 'a third of your body weight in stone as litres of water each day', so in your case you should be drinking at least 3.5 litres of water each day and about one level teaspoon of salt.

Patient: That's a lot.

Me: It seems like that at first, but give it a go. Work up to it over the next couple of weeks. I do recommend a nice drink of salted water at least once or twice per day, preferably in the morning and evening, but the most important thing to do is get the ratio correct.

(I take out a teaspoon and put a level amount of salt in it, then pour it into my hand) This is how much salt you should ideally be consuming each day. You can put some on your food, some in your water and even just take a small pinch from time to time if you feel like it.

Patient: It's as simple as that?

Me: Yes, (I point to a litre bottle of water) as long as you are drinking the equivalent of three of these bottles each day as well, you'll start to get properly hydrated and most likely start to feel like a new person very quickly.

Patient: But I've never drunk that much of water each day in my life!

Me: It's OK, that's normal, most of us are chronically dehydrated and we don't even know it because we lost the ability to recognise thirst, probably a long time ago. Increase the amount of water you drink incrementally over the next week or two. Look at the old folk walking in the streets, they are so completely dehydrated, you can see the pain on their faces, do you want to end up like that?

Patient: No way, I already feel much older than I am.

Me: So drink the water and take the salt, and do it religiously for a while. Don't 'forget' to drink water and take salt. If a little voice in your head says 'drink some water' act on it straight away, don't put it off until later. If another little voice in your head replies 'You don't need to drink water now, you can drink some later', ignore it!

Patient: I quite like herbal tea, is that the same?

Me: Yes, but green tea has some caffeine in it as well, so don't use that to rehydrate. Put your herbal tea bag in a large glass, fill it to the top and refill it if necessary. You can enjoy the occasional cup of normal tea, but not habitually, not 5 or 6 cups per day, that's far too much.

Patient: I've drunk tea since I was a kid, how much can I have?

Me: I suggest 2 cups per day maximum, lowering it to 1 cup per day after a while. You see, a plant creates caffeine in order to keep predators off it, it is a poison and according to studies, for every cup of tea you drink, you pee out 1.4 cups of water, so you need to compensate by drinking even more water afterwards.

Patient: That's very interesting; my doctor never told me that.

Me: That's because doctors don't learn it at medical college. They are taught that 'dry mouth is the first sign of dehydration in the body' which is a reversal of the truth; actually it is one of the last. They don't even learn the difference between the real salt and the table salt.

Patient: He just says that my condition is incurable and that I need to take anti-inflammatory drugs.

Me: Well, I'm telling you different. Do you know what the cartilage is?

Patient: Yes, it's what keeps the bones from rubbing against each other.

Me: Do you know what it is primarily made of?

Patient: No.

Me: Water and salt! It's no wonder your joints are aching. You have to get your water and salt levels corrected. It will only get worse if you don't.

Patient: But I was never told that, it's amazing!

Me: You'll find that your cartilage begins to rebuild itself along with loads of other benefits which you can read about in Dr.Batmaghelidj's book if you have the time. Either way, drink the water and salt.

Patient: I will.

Me: Also, you should know that when the body is dehydrated and salt deficient, as yours is, it tries to cope by involuntarily squeezing the colon walls to squeeze the pooh and extract moisture and minerals from it. This 'pooh water' then seeps through the colon walls and is reintroduced into the body, into the lungs, heart, brain etc. You don't want pooh water pumping around your body, do you?

Patient: No way. I was never told that.

Me: There's no money in this kind of advice, that's why it doesn't see the light of the day much, but it's true and it's serious. There are lots of nutritionists and natural therapists that aren't aware of it either. Arthritis isn't the only effect of dehydration, loads of other diseases such as asthma and even cancer are either caused by it or exasperated by it, it's a world problem!

Patient: I think, I'll read that book you were talking about.

Me: Good idea, we also have some photocopied information; you can take away with you.

Patient: Thanks.

Me: So, I've told you about the first two parts of the Five Point

Plan, water and salt. Try it out for a couple of weeks and let me know how you are getting on when you next see me. The other parts of the plan are urine therapy, diet and exercise but we'll deal with them when we have more time.

Patient: Urine? Do I have to drink my urine?

Me: No you don't. It is amazing to drink it but you don't have to. I swear by it but it's probably not essential for you. As far as your diet is concerned, for now, just try to avoid too much junk food and eat plenty of fruits and vegetables. I'll give you a sheet to take away with you.

Patient: OK, thanks very much.

Me: Also, here - have a free pouch of French Atlantic sea salt to get you started, we give free pouches of salt to anyone who wants them.

Patient: Great! That makes it easy.

Me: That's the idea! Natural healthcare doesn't have to be complicated. Stick to the plan, get hydrated, get your salt level more corrected and I look forward to hearing about your progress soon.

SECOND CONVERSATION: DIET
(Four munutes)

Me: Hi, so how are you feeling now?

Patient: A lot better actually. I think the water and salt is really helping.

Me: And your joints?

Patient: They are improving for sure, I'm feeling less pain than when I last saw you.

Me: Excellent, how about your energy levels?

Patient: I hadn't actually thought about it but yes, I feel like I've got more energy recently.

Me: Great, that's because you're getting all re-hydrated! Have you been sticking to the WaterCure?

Patient: Oh yes, and I've read all the pamphlets you gave me.

Me: Did you like them?

Patient: Yes, I photocopied a couple of them and gave them to my mother.

Me: Good, so how much water are you drinking these days?

Patient: Over three litres each day like you said.

Me: And the salt?

Patient: Yes, I'm putting some in my water bottles and putting a bit on my food.

Me: Do you feel like continuing with the WaterCure programme?

Patient: Definitely!

Me: Good. OK, let's talk about your diet. What sort of food do you eat for breakfast?

Patient: Cereal usually, sometimes toast as well. And a cup of tea.

Me: Do you add milk and sugar to your cereal?

Patient: Yes.

Me: Regular milk and sugar from the supermarket?

Patient: Um, yes.

Me: And for lunch?

Patient: Well, I'm usually at work, so I have a sandwich and some crisps or a chocolate bar.

Me: White bread with margarine?

Patient: Yes, I prefer white bread.

Me: What do you drink with your lunch?

Patient: A can of cola or something like that.

Me: OK, and for supper?

Patient: It depends how busy I am. Sometimes I cook for myself, sometimes I get a take-away or go to a café.

Me: What sort of food do you prepare for yourself?

Patient: Well, nothing too complicated. Sausages and mashed potato, pasta with some chicken and sauce...I like the pre-prepared food from Waitrose (supermarket) as well.

Me: And if you get a take-away...what sort do you like?

Patient: Usually a Chinese, sometimes I get a pizza or kebab, something like that.

Me: OK, I'm taking a note of all this. How often do you eat organic food?

Patient: Um, not really sure. I don't spend money on the expensive stuff in the supermarkets if that's what you mean?

Me: Well, yes but you can get organic produce delivered from the local farm much cheaper. OK, so let's recap on the basis of your diet. Pasteurised non-organic milk, refined white sugar, refined bleached white bread, refined margarine, mechanically re-claimed meat, chemical sugar rich soft drinks, meat, pasta,

Chinese take-away. It doesn't sound good, does it?

Patient: Well, not when you put it like that. But I do buy vegetables from the supermarket sometimes.

Me: How often?

Patient: Oh, um…well, I usually eat the pre-prepared meals – they have vegetables in them. I do buy onions and tomatoes sometimes, if I make my own pasta sauces.

Me: That's not nearly good enough, I'm afraid. The good news is that considering you already feel better from going on the WaterCure, you're going to feel marvellous when you change your diet. The bad news is that your body is currently chock-a-block, full of poisonous left-over material from all the rubbish you've been eating.

Patient: Oh. But I've eaten like that for ages…

Me: Which is why you're sitting here in front of me looking for a way to feel better?

Patient: Yes, of course. So what do you suggest?

Me: I really think you need to go back to nature more often. Relish natural foods and enjoy them for what they are. You'll learn what you need to know in the pamphlets so I won't go into much detail now, suffice to say all this refined food has to drastically cut down and replaced with whole food.

Patient: But that means spending all my life in the kitchen and learning complicated recipes!

Me: Who says?

Patient: Well, it does…doesn't it?

Me: It can be so if you want, but it can also be very quick and easy. I'm a bachelor and I don't like spending too much time in the kitchen and washing up. I'll tell you something important now; the secret is really in eating raw, organic vegetarian food. Salads for instance…they can be really nice if you use quality ingredients and make them properly. Don't turn your nose up! Trust me, the salads you've tried in the past have probably been terrible, people in this country don't know about salads. You can't mix a few poor quality vegetables together and expect a nice salad. Anyway, I suggest you look at the information and recipes and just try it. Just try for a few weeks by replacing some of the bread, meat, cheese, take-away etc. judiciously with wholesome, organic salads. Think of food as medicine, just for now and I swear you'll be glad you did by the time you next see me.

Patient: You make it sound good. So, I have to change my diet completely?

Me: Not really. Yes, cut out the refined sugar – but you can replace it with a bit of honey or some unrefined sugar that you can get in the whole food shop. Keep on with the cereal if you really like it, just buy an organic version and use organic soya/almond/rice milk instead, the naturally sweetened versions are actually very tasty I think. Alternatively, I would recommend not to eat anything in the morning and have a long fruit or vegetable juice and, say a pint of hot water with some salt, apple cider vinegar and molasses. It tastes fine, fills you up and gives loads of energy. The recipes for all this are in the information sheets.

I would say try to cut out all meat if you possibly can, it will only harm you in the long run. If that sounds too hard, stick to eating some fresh fish once in a while but as for chicken sandwiches, Chinese take-away and kebabs…well, that's a big no-no, sorry… I have to say stop it, at least for a few weeks so you can see how you feel.

Patient: OK, I'll give it a go. I just can't afford to spend lots of money.

Me: You won't. You'll save quite a lot on what you don't spend on pre-packaged food, take-away and meat. That money can be re-allocated to getting hold of decent quality veggies etc.

Patient: Alright, I'll try it.

Me: Read the information and be enthusiastic about eating naturally if you can.

Patient: Now you're really pushing the envelope!

Me: Why not? I'm right you know, a natural diet really does taste better than an artificial one...

Patient: OK! I try it for sure and let you know how I get on.

Me: Excellent. You know you can always email or call if you have any questions.

Patient: Yes, thanks.

Me: Three weeks, OK? Be disciplined.

Patient: I promise.

THIRD CONVERSATION: EXERCISE
(Five minutes)

Me: Hi, you're looking much better! How do you feel?

Patient: Thanks, I feel much better. I've been following the advice pretty much to the letter and I must say it's making the world of difference.

Me: That's excellent news. You're following the WaterCure fine?

Patient: Yes.

Me: 100% sure?

Patient: Um, nearly. I've not had much salt in the last few days, not sure why.

Me: Do you feel any aversion to the salt?

Patient: No, I like it. I guess I've just forgotten to take it recently.

Me: No problem, but do make sure to make a stronger commitment to correcting your salt levels from now on, ok?

Patient: Yes, sure.

Me: So, is there anything more you want to talk about the WaterCure?

Patient: No, I don't think so.

Me: There's loads of information on the Internet websites, I list on the sheet I gave you last time; if you want more information, or just ask me sometime.

Patient: Ok. I've been reading some of the watercure.com website.

Me: Interesting?

Patient: Sure.

Me: And how about the diet? Is everything going ok. There?

Patient: Yes for sure. I've been quite disciplined with it all.

Me: Good. So let's talk about exercise for a while. I can see you could do with losing a bit of weight.

Patient: Definitely. I have actually lost some weight since I last saw you.

Me: My guess is that you've been eating less because of being on the WaterCure?

Patient: Yes I think so. I don't feel so hungry generally.

Me: That's because your body knows it is getting all re-hydrated! If your body could talk it would probably say something like 'thanks a lot mate, I need this!'

Patient: It feels like it is saying something like that actually!

Me: So, in terms of physical fitness, how would you describe yourself?

Patient: Hmmm, lazy I think. I suppose you could say my life is pretty sedentary.

Me: How old are you now?

Patient: Fourty-six.

Me: And when would you say you were last in good physical shape?

Patient: Oh dear, um…probably not since I was thirty. I got my job that I've still got now and well, I just haven't been that interesting in going to the gym or whatever.

Me: Sixteen years of neglect eh? Doesn't sound too good, does it?

Patient: (Laughs) not when you put it like that, no!

Me: You're physically lazy! You've already told me that. It's ok. But you have neglected yourself for a long time. Do you know that?

Patient: Yes, I suppose I have.

Me: I'm sure you have and I'm telling you like this, so you move beyond it, defeat the dragon, so to speak.

Patient: No, you're right. I need a push.

Me: Ok, exercise is really important. If you don't move the body, take deep breathes, break into a sweat, get the blood pumping on a regular basis you're going to suffer, especially in old age.

Patient: Like my mum, I don't want to end up like that.

Me: Like many people's mums:...and dads. Most people are not getting nearly enough exercise. How willing are you to get more physically active in your life?

Patient: I know I've got to do it.

Me: Good, so come on, how willing are you to do more exercise?

Patient: Well, the truth is, I don't really like it. I've never liked sports or going to the gym or jogging and all that stuff.

Me: Not even when you were a kid?

Patient: Well, when I was much younger I suppose, yes, I guess I loved running around and all that kind of thing.

Me: See, you loved it. Why do you think you loved it then and now you don't?

Patient: Um, well, I was a kid, I had lots of energy.

Me: So even rigorous exercise seemed quite easy.

Patient: Yes, I suppose it was.

Me: Did you know you can have that kind energy back again if you want it?

Patient: That would be good...but I'm forty six, I'm overweight...

Me: And you're being defeatist!

Patient: (Laughs) Ok, I know I would like to have lots of energy so what's your advice?

Me: Well, I would say start slow and gentle. We want this to be a pleasant transition. I think it's important for you to get the blood pumping each day, even if it's just for a few minutes to begin with.

Patient: Please don't tell me I have to go jogging!

Me: No, not if you don't want to. You don't even have to leave your house if you don't want, but I think it will be good for you to breathe some fresh air and get some sunlight. Do you like walking?

Patient: Not really!

Me: Do you think you could get to like walking?

Patient: Maybe.

Me: Well, try it sometime. Don't be in a hurry, just go for walk somewhere you like and take a few deep breaths, ok?

Patient: Ok, I'll try it.

Me: Try to get into a pattern of some sort. I know it's hard with work and all the other things, but I'm sure you can find time. Stretch the legs, take deep breaths, relax your body, catch some sunlight on your skin…and enjoy it! Ok?

Patient: I'll try.

Me: Don't try…do! Don't try to enjoy yourself…enjoy yourself. Walking is nice, look around, give a think about your life, fill your lungs…it's nice! Don't try.

Patient: (Laughs) Ok.

Me: So how many times do you plan to go walking in the next week?

Patient: Do you think I should go every day?

Me: What do you think?

Patient: It could be good.

Me: Yes, some exercise each and every day is very important. If for some reason going for a walk isn't possible, then do some exercise indoors. It's very easy actually; you just need to know a few basic warm-ups and stretches. Here are a few sheets with some ideas to get you started.

Patient: Thanks.

Me: There are about six warm-up exercises and I think 8 basic stretches to work with. You can do them in front of the TV if you want, it doesn't really matter for now. Just…try to enjoy it…or at least don't do this stuff begrudgingly…you know what I mean?

Patient: Yes. You mean I've got to get into it properly.

Me: You have to re-learn how to enjoy exercising again. It's great because as you progress each day, slowly-slowly, as you overcome laziness and all those negative little voices…it gets better and better! Really it does, week after week you'll feel stronger and stronger…happier I promise. Do you think you can commit to enjoying, say at least twenty minutes of exercise each day, whether that is brisk walking or warm-ups or whatever?

Patient: Sure.

Me: Now, don't push it with these stretches. Just relax and breathe gently, like it says on the sheets. Remember that you are going to be working muscles that probably haven't been worked for years, the last thing you want at this stage is to pull a muscle or get all achy, and then give up with it all, ok?

Patient: Sure.

Me: Have you got twenty minutes free later?

Patient: Yes.

Me: Good, so go on a nice walk, do a few warm ups and stretches if you want as well, but get the blood pumping and have a good think about what you want to achieve, in terms of health. You know it's important.

Patient: And long overdue. Thanks for pushing me, I need it. My wife tells me sometimes, but it's good to have someone from the outside to tell me straight…

Me: That's what I'm here for, it's my pleasure really.

Patient: Thanks.

Me: Thank me by telling me next time that you are getting into a regular exercise routine, that's what I want you to say and judging by the way you've worked so well on the WaterCure and the diet…well, I think you'll really get into it once your body has got used to the change. It won't take long, just commit to, say two weeks to begin with. Two weeks of daily exercise, give it a fair crack of the whip, enjoy it and tell me how you feel next time I see you, ok?

Patient: Sure.

FOURTH CONVERSATION: URINE THERAPY
(Five minutes)

Me: Hello again, how are you today?

Patient: I feel ok, thanks.

Me: So, it's been a couple of weeks since I last saw you, what have you been up to?

Patient: Well, I had a slight 'relapse' for a few days…I got a bit depressed and resorted to my old habits, take away food etc, but I'm back on track now.

Me: Not to worry, how is your exercise going generally?

Patient: It's ok, I've been walking most days along the sea front.

Me: Is it ok?

Patient: Yes, I'm getting more used to it now.

Me: Do you feel the benefits yet?

Patient: Yes I think I do. People are saying I'm looking healthier and that kind of stuff.

Me: So, what kind of benefits do you feel?

Patient: Just an all-round thing really, um…I am losing weight for sure.

Me: That's good news. You still seem a bit down.

Patient: Yes, I don't know why, the last few days I've felt unsure about a few things.

Me: To do with your health plan?

Patient: Oh no, I'm pleased with all that. I'm not sure what is wrong exactly, emotional stuff…just feel a bit naggy…

Me: Well, that's ok, it will pass. Do you feel things are changing in your life?

Patient: Kind of, I'm changing - I know that.

Me: Change can be hard. But you're happy with your health?

Patient: Definitely. I'm actually quite enthusiastic about it. I don't drink any of that sugary stuff any more at all and still drinking lots of water.

Me: What did you eat yesterday?

Patient: Umm…a fruit salad with yoghurt for breakfast.

Me: Nice?

Patient: Yes

Me: Organic fruit?

Patient: Yes, apart from the bananas, my organic ones are still green at the moment.

Me: No problem, at least it wasn't a bacon sandwich!

Patient: Oh no, I can't face that kind of thing any more.

Me: So, what else did you eat yesterday?

Patient: A sandwich at lunch, I know it's not so healthy, but it wasn't a meaty one.

Me: Well, ok. White bread and Margarine.

Patient: Well, yes. The selection of food at work isn't great.

Me: So don't waste your money on it. Really, try to get to a point where that kind of food doesn't even tempt you, ok?

Patient: Yes ok. Normally I skip lunch and have something at home at about seven.

Me: There's loads of things you can take into work to nibble on if you get hungry. Bananas, nuts, humus, carrots…

Patient: I know, they call it 'rabbit food' at work.

Me: Well, that's there problem. Are these people healthy and happy?

Patient: No!

Me: So ignore them. Anyway, we need to learn a few lessons from the animals about how to feed ourselves.

Patient: (Laughs) that's true!

Me: And your evening meal?

Patient: It's good. Like it says in the sheets, I made a big salad and kept it airtight in the fridge. I have a big portion with whatever else I am eating…not burgers or anything anymore, yes, it's fine, I like it actually.

Me: So you mentioned you'd been eating takeaways because you were feeling down. How was that?

Patient: Crap. I ate the food and every time felt worse afterwards and just wanted to go to sleep.

Me: What was it – Pizza, Chinese?

Patient: Yes.

Me: It's alright, don't beat yourself up over it – the junk food will do all that for you!

Patient: Yes…I actually felt sick one time.

Me: It's ok to lapse sometimes, it's natural but it won't help you, I guess you know that now.

Patient: Yes, I don't think I'll order pizza again for quite a while; I ate a large one to myself and felt ill.

Me: Yuk, I think I would too. But you're back on the straight and narrow now? You want to keep on with the programme?

Patient: Definitely. It's what I need.

Me: And you mentioned that you were interested in the information about urine therapy.

Patient: Well, yes. It did sound very interesting. Do you think it could really help me out?

Me: I do. I've had a great success with urine therapy in my own life and can recommend it for you as well.

Patient: Do you drink it?

Me: Yes, most of the mornings I have about half a cup full from my copper cup, I keep in the bathroom.

Patient: (Makes a face)…it just seems a bit disgusting.

Me: I know it does at first. I was challenged to try it about six years ago and I pulled a similar face as you! But you know I never looked back.

Patient: So what do you recommend?

Me: Well, you say you're still following the WaterCure…

Patient: Yes.

Me: So that means your urine is fairly clear right?

Patient: Yes, I've noticed that.

Me: You know why your urine used to be a darker yellow in colour?

Patient: Well, 'cos I was dehydrated I think.

Me: Yes, you see when the body is dehydrated, it subconsciously squeezes moisture from the pooh in the colon, which then seeps through the colon walls and pumps all around your body… around the brain, through the kidneys etc.

Patient: Urgh…

Me: Yes, it's pretty gross. Anyway, the thing to remember is this: the closer to the colour of pooh that your pee is, the more 'faecal extracted' the moisture in your body is.

Patient: Right, I'll remember that.

Me: So, what I'm trying to say is that your urine won't taste bad, ok?

Patient: Oh good.

Me: Yes, it will be strange at first. It's something you've probably never done before…

Patient: Actually, my mum said she used to find me drinking out of my potty sometimes!

Me: That happens a lot. Very young kids seem quite happy to drink and play around with urine actually. But in my opinion… and this has been going on since ancient time…why not? Urine is not a waste product like people say. Pooh is a waste product… I'm not advocating that anyone eat their pooh…

Patient: Good!

Me: But really, urine is a highly refined form of our own blood. People say 'oh, you can't drink that, the body is getting rid of it 'cos it is toxic, how can it be healthy to drink it' but I'm sure they've got it wrong.

Patient: That's what my wife says, but after I read the information, it seemed quite logical actually.

Me: It is logical. There's loads of ways to explain it. One way is to think of it as a bio-feedback-stimulator….it's like…whatever is wrong with you, whatever imbalance there is…the information is contained in your urine. Like when you go for a pee, a CD ROM is coming out of you with all the information on it. Then you put the CD ROM into the computer – your mouth – and the body says 'oh right, that's the problem'. Does that make sense?

Patient: Yes, a bit like a vaccination.

Me: Yes. The best vaccine in my opinion and free as well. But it's more than that, they've found well over a thousand beneficial ingredients – minerals, enzymes etc – it's really loaded with so much goodness, if you could split it up and make all the ingredients into tablets you make a fortune every time you go to the loo!

Patient: Yes?

Me: You'd be surprised how much of these 'miracle' drugs contain human urine, urea is amazing for the skin, the pharmaceutical companies pay the 'port-a–loo' people for the human urine that is collected and then extracted for some of the goodness to sell at massively inflated prices to people with skin problems.

Patient: Ha, typical!

Me: Anyway, what I was saying is that these various supplements that cost so much, really it's much better to just drink a little urine each morning in most cases. As long as you're not living a seriously toxic, acidic life – or taking hard drugs or something, a little sip of urine each morning can work wonders.

Patient: I just seems so weird!

Me: Well, most people don't do it – but many wise people do, especially in the east – three million in china, I read, and it's very popular in India too.

Patient: Yes, I read the old prime minister drank it, that was very interesting.

Me: Moraji Desai you mean?

Patient: Yes.

Me: He really was a great example to the Indian people. He actually had the conviction to stand up and say to them – 'Yes,

I drink urine. Yes, I live hygienically…and you should too!' Can you imagine Tony Blair saying something like that?

Patient: No! Or George Bush!

Me: India is a very special country. So, if you really don't like the idea of swallowing, you know you can actually benefit greatly from just swilling it around under the tongue for five or ten seconds and then spitting it out.

Patient: Yes, I read something about that.

Me: Yes, it programs the lymph which is concentrated under the tongue which in turn sends the message throughout the whole lymphatic network around the body.

Patient: That's quite powerful when you think about it.

Me: I know, I think it's amazing.

Patient: But if I put it in my mouth, I think I'll swallow it anyway, I don't really care, it just seems strange.

Me: Ok, it's good you want to try it, I think you'll look back and feel glad you did. It's not essential, but do you have a copper cup you can use?

Patient: No.

Me: It's ok, you can use a mug or glass or something. If you see a copper cup in a shop, you might want to buy it. They say copper is the best vessel to drink from; it has the similar frequency to urine.

Patient: I think I can find a copper cup; I'll look in the antique shops.

Me: So, the morning pee is the best. It has had plenty of time to 'brew' in the body, it also contains important bio chemicals such as serotonin and melatonin, chemicals that are said to be produced during our dream.

Patient: Interesting.

Me: But if you don't drink it in the morning for some reason, you can drink it any time. Less than half a cup is fine, 50ml... less. Just make sure you hold it under your tongue for a few seconds.

Patient: And that's it?

Me: Yes, I mean you can use it for loads of stuff. I wash my hair with it, sometimes I drink a lot in one day, maybe a litre or so, but usually I find that my morning sip is enough. Just make sure you brush your teeth afterwards, ok?

Patient: Sure! I guess it can make the breath smell.

Me: Yes, I've known a couple of people who got so keen on urine therapy they smelt of it a bit, like a tramp had turned up in the room but I couldn't see him!

Patient: Gross.

Me: So that's it, have a sip in the morning before you brush your teeth.

Patient: I'll start tomorrow.

Most of the consultations I held followed a very similar pattern and invariably, those patients who followed the advice showed great all-round improvements.

ACCOUNT FROM MARIA, GOA, 2006

'James, let me thank you for the simple advice you gave me. This MS which I have developed since I was 15 years old, effectively after my first teeth amalgam fillings hasn't let me one week without pain since 5 years. Since my daughter Norangel was born I have been very busy, too much pressure and I have been feeling very depressed because of the continuous increase of the disease.

I manage this unbalance, step after step with a better diet, complementary therapies, acupuncture, tibetan and aryuvedic stuff, belief, peace of mind development, energy work and so on...Now, since meeting you I am so pleased to discover the Five Point Plan, such a simple and powerful way to make my body lighter. Since the day I began to drink far more water and with real sea salt, I felt even the next morning, an amelioration, more fresh body. After 5 days, I rediscover some fine sensitivity in my feet and hands. The Spirulina now gives my system all the vitamins and minerals it needs and the colloidal silver solved in 24 hours the mouth infection I had when I met you. It is great that I get a direct positive observation of its effects, so I drink it everyday with lot of trust and my body likes it! Thank you again James and let us keep in touch for some even better news: 1, 2, 3 ...weeks without pain. Everyday a new life opens. All the best to you and to each person who is in need of new hope. There is!'

MY RESPONSE TO MARIA'S ACCOUNT:

I met Maria in Goa and she said she had Multiple Sclerosis. I noticed straight away that she was dehydrated by looking at her eyes and skin. I asked her how much water she drank and wasn't surprised when she answered 'not much, maybe 1 or 2 glasses per day'. After a couple of years of working with MS, Cancer, AIDS and Arthritis patients in London, I came to the conclusion that it is very often unintentional chronic dehydration that leads to disease in the body. I also found a strong correlation between auto-immune diseases such as MS and amalgam/mercury fillings.

In 2003, I gave a talk to members and coordinators of the Multiple Sclerosis Society in London, in which I explained my findings, which are summarized below:

> ➢ There is no 'one cure' for MS. It is often a mixture of diet

and lifestyle problems.

> Taking drugs such as 'Interferon' do not address the cause of the problem. (One lady in the audience told me she took over 50 tablets each day!).

> Everyone in the audience (around 60 people) was chronically dehydrated.

> Amalgam/mercury fillings can be very dangerous to health and should be removed correctly.

> Hempseed oil, whole food diet, pure water, pure sea salt, colloidal silver, spirulina and gentle yoga-style exercises can drastically help MS sufferers.

> Unlike many people who have suffered diseases such as MS for many years, Maria had been given all sorts of advice over the years from alternative healers and doctors, but no one had looked at the most important factor, which is related to rectifying the hydration and salt deficiency.

> The primary focus of the Five Point plan is the work of Dr. Batmaghelidj, Hygienic whole food nutrition and yoga practices, including urine therapy. When practiced together they provide a particularly powerful and simple way to attain health and well-being.

WHY DIAGNOSIS IS NOT DEEMED SO IMPORTANT IN THE FIVE POINT PLAN

The diagnosis is a man made art which the inherent intelligence of the body is not concerned with. Dr Herbert Shelton was a prominent Natural Hygienist who correctly said that diagnosis is the least important part of getting well.

There are so many different systems of diagnosis, including:

> Medical

> Ayurvedic
> Traditional Chinese (meridians),
> Iridiagnosis (studying the iris)
> Naturopathic
> X-ray
> Applied kinesiology
> Pulse and tongue diagnosis
> Germ theory
> Virus theory
> Genetics

Yet I feel that all these systems, however ancient, are overlooking the most important fact of illness, that all bodily parts and cells are affected at the same time, with the weakest part manifesting first, followed by the next weakest.

The enervation / toxemia / deficiency cycle

All human life has a blood stream, which nourishes the body and removes disease causing germs. Life force/prana/chi is ubiquitous and when the body is allowed to sufficient rest, sunlight, nutrition etc the same power that created the body will also heal the body; all the rest is 'jazz'.

Aside from injuries, emergencies or complications resulting from injury, diseases are caused by any or all of just three factors as follows:

> Deficiency
> Enervation
> Toxemia

The deficiency of necessary food substances (such as

carbohydrates, proteins, fats, minerals, vitamins and enzymes) leads to breakdown of cells, tissues and organs. The modern medicine gives names to the various diseases according to the particular location of the breakdown.

The enervation refers to the weakening of vital nerve energy (through stress, tiredness, negative thoughts, over eating etc).

There are 2 sources of toxemia:

➢ Toxic foods / drinks

➢ Toxic chemicals

Retention of this excess leads to decomposition of the food and the production of irritating and toxic chemical waste. This waste provides fertile ground for the growth of microbes and other various species of bacteria, which further increase the intensity of the toxic state.

Dr. John Tilden formulated the enervation/toxemia model as a recurring cycle whereby the body can encounter any number of diseases over its lifespan.

Without any diagnosis, the principles of the Five Point Plan have shown time and time again to bring about true health and healing. Following the WaterCure and cleaning up diet / lifestyle habits is very often all that is needed for a full recovery in a short space of time; no diagnostic labels necessary.

The animals know this intuitively and it is high time that we humans become aware of it consciously.

The ideal way to treat patients is to use whatever diagnostic knowledge is available, but not to be overly concerned with the accuracy of it.

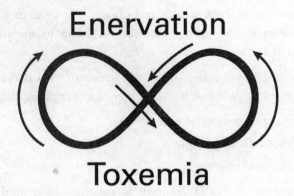

Enervation

Toxemia

'The job of the healer is amuse the patient whilst nature does the healing.'

- Chinese saying

WATER

'The information on dehydration is ground-breaking. The explanation I have been able to put together will educate the public about dehydration. And basically, it will turn everyone into a healer of their own bodies. And they, in turn, become healers for others around them. This is how information is spread so far.'

-Dr. Fereydoon Batmanghelidj

Introduction

Dehydration can be defined as:

1. The process of removing water from a substance or compound.

2. The excessive loss of water from the body or from an organ or body part, as from illness or fluid deprivation.

Water is one of the most important element on earth and without it life would very quickly cease to exist. A key factor that makes for a healthier, happier, longer life is, drinking enough pure water every day. Seeing as the body is comprising of over 70% water, it makes sense to keep that water clean by regularly flushing it through new supplies. The vast majority of us are ignoring this priceless health tip and needlessly suffering as a result.

Moreover, it is quite shocking to think that when the body is dehydrated it resorts to obtaining moisture from the stagnated, compacted faecal matter lurking in the colon. This causes constipation and leads to a state of auto-intoxication (or toxemia), which refers to the pollution of the blood by allowing the development of a cesspool in the guts. None of us want to have excrement-obtained water pumping through our brain, lungs, kidneys and other internal organs yet this is precisely what is happening when we neglect our body's many cries for water. Our heart disease, cancer, headaches, acne, allergies, diabetes and arthritis are just some of the many problems that can stem from this dehydration.

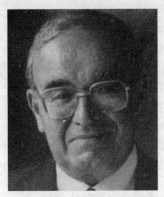

Fig. 2.1 Dr. Batmanghelidj

'WaterCure' pioneer Dr. Batmanghelidj provides powerful evidence to illustrate that many of the 'diseases of unknown etiology (origin)' are primarily caused by chronic dehydration. On his informative website www.watercure.com he overviews the 'tragedy' of not recognising this fact in a concise, logical and hard-hitting way.

He reasons that modern medical science is built on four major mistakes:

> 'Dry mouth is the only sign of dehydration'. In 1764, Albrecht von Haller first claimed dry mouth as a sign of thirst. This view was supported by Walter Bradford Cannon in 1918 and since then this erroneous belief has altered the course of medicine and skewed the medical profession's understanding of bodily water regulation. In truth, dry

mouth is one of the very last signs of dehydration, coming after a whole host of other symptoms.

> 'Water is a simple substance that only dissolves and circulates different things'. Actually water is not a simple, inert substance at all. It serves both life-sustaining functions (as acknowledged by medical science) and life-giving functions.

> 'The human body can regulate effectively its water intake throughout the life span of the person'. In truth, our drought perception ability usually diminishes with age – older people frequently fail to recognise that they need to drink water.

> 'Any fluid can replace the water needs of the body'. The manufactured beverages do not function in the same pristine way as pure water does and are often diuretic, signifying that they serve to further dehydrate the body.

ARTHRITIS AND JOINT PAIN

"Conventional doctors will tell you the only way to treat arthritis is with over-the-counter pain relievers, including aspirin, Tylenol®, and NSAIDs like Advil®. But long-term use can put you at a risk for potentially lethal side effects; for example, gastrointestinal bleeding, liver damage and kidney failure. Even nutritional supplements like glucosamine and chondroitin sulphate fail to treat the true source of your pain, and simply don't work for everyone.

Whenever you feel pain in any of your joints, the first thought that should occur to you is, 'My body is severely short of water." That's because the parts of your body that suffer most when you are dehydrated are those without direct vascular circulation, like joint cartilage. Because of lack of sufficient water and the nourishment that water provides, cartilage cells eventually shrivel up and die. Taking medications to mask the pain simply allows you to put more wear and tear on your joints, making matters worse. Only water can restore your joints to its more youthful strength and flexibility.'

- Dr. Batmanghelidj

I was so impressed with this paragraph that inspired me to make a small poster of it and displayed it in the window of my local newsagent. I offered free information and a free pouch of high quality sea salt to anyone who was interested. The result was disappointing. The town has around 60% OAP population and I could see people on the streets everyday who were suffering joint pain yet after two months of displaying the advert, nobody phoned also for the free WaterCure pack. It reminds me of the saying 'we all stumble across the truth sometimes in our lives yet most of us pick ourselves up, brush ourselves down and carry like nothing had happened.' If only these arthritic folk would realise that water and salt alone can rebuild cartilage. On the positive side, a few months later I did manage to get a three-page feature about Urine Therapy and the WaterCure in the local newspaper, so hopefully more people paid attention to that.

The unintentional chronic dehydration leads to many pains in the body which are either locally registered or central nervous system registered. In the earlier stages of dehydration, pain killers can mask local pain signals however it is only a matter of time before the brain becomes the direct centre for monitoring the pain perpetuation until hydration is resumed. Compelling evidence shows that in many cases, the occurrence of pain is in reality a 'drought crisis management signal'. One way of looking at it could be that the intelligence of the body creates pain in a desperate attempt to force the 'personality' to drink more water.

In his ground-breaking paper 'Neurotransmitter Histamine, An

Alternative Viewpoint', Dr. Batmanghelidj reveals the purpose and function of histamine in the body as a water regulator.

The basic gist of the paper is that histamine will act as a temporary substitute for water in a dehydrated body by providing energy for some highly sensitive body functions, such as respiration or neurotransmission.

MORE THAN 'JUST ANOTHER HEALING SYSTEM'

Whilst I am aware that many practitioners mention the importance of drinking enough water each day to patients, few are actually aware of exactly how important it is to get the water and salt ratio perfectly balanced. The WaterCure is not 'just another healing system'; it is the backbone of health itself. This is why Dr. Batmanghelidj was so passionate about his work; because he knew that the vast majority of medical doctors, natural therapists and the general public were unaware of the core importance of water and salt in relation to health. Thanks to his ground-breaking work, myself and many other people are now aware of this simple truth.

It is important to drink water steadily throughout the day and it is equally important that the body is fully capable of retaining the water. A regular intake of real salt (which contains up to 85 minerals) and some whole food once in a while will make the world of difference as far as mineral deficiency and related illnesses are concerned, however salt also enables the water we drink to permeate in our cells through it's osmotic function. To put it simply; if the body is lacking salt the water will not get into the cells and we will become dehydrated at the cellular level. There are two 'lakes' in the human body. The first one is the lake that the cells swim in and the second is the lake that is found inside each and every cell. In order for these cells to remain hydrated and 'plum like', salt must be present in the blood.

The guidelines vary as to how much water we should be drinking according to our particular needs and situations, however less than two litres throughout the day is generally not advisable. For many, especially those who are actively aiming to detoxify their body, double this quantity is recommended. Have a long drink of water in the morning and keep drinking through the day, perhaps remembering to drink every time you urinate. If your urine is a dark yellow colour, the chances are that you are dehydrated. The closer to the colour of faeces that your urine is, the more auto-intoxicated you are becoming. With this in mind, it is advisable to treat dehydration seriously and be good to yourself with regular drinks of pure water.

I haven't met many people who are actually getting the correct hydration each day. In his book 'Life Flow One, The Solution For Heart Disease' Karl Loren writes about the results of his research into exactly how much pure water people are generally drinking each day:

'Let's consider a glass of water to be about eight ounces. It should be considered, also, plain! No flavourings, no fizzy bubbles. It could be from the tap, bottle or through a filter. But, it is plain water and you drink it down, in sips or large swallows -- but down it goes -- plain water -- with or without food.

> There will be about 10% who never drink a plain glass of water during the day. They have justifications, such as the orange juice, coffee or milk they drink.

> There will be about 30% who drink one or two glasses per day.

> There will be about 40% who drink three to five glasses per day.

> There will be about 15% who drink six to nine glasses per day.

> There will be about 5% who drink ten or more glasses per day.'

Don't wait until you are physically uncomfortable with dehydration, before you have a drink.

A closer look at water

'I have found that distilled water is a sovereign remedy for my rheumatism. I attribute my almost perfect health largely to distilled water.'

- Alexander Bell

Wouldn't it be nice if we could just turn on the tap and drink safe, healthy water whenever we wanted? Unfortunately, it is not as simple as that. Generally our water supply is a prime factor for illness in the world so if you are still drinking it; you should take cautious steps to purify it or drink a healthier, less toxic variety of water instead. The tap waters around the world differ according to local restrictions; what is legal and acceptable in some countries is illegal in others. In America, for instance, fluoride is found in tap water where as in most of the UK this wicked ingredient is banned. That's not to say UK tap water is good, it is not.

There are thousands of chemical compounds in our tap water from industry, agriculture and domestic homes. Tap water drinkers ingest small dose of these chemicals every day and no one knows for sure what the long-term effects may be. Industrial chemical waste found in landfills is a major cause of water pollution as is radioactive waste and runoff pesticides from agricultural areas. A particularly nasty ingredient that is added to tap water is chlorine, which is found in UK tap water. These additives are big business for those that make and supply them to the water companies however the effect they have on health can be devastating.

A FEW EXAMPLES OF WHAT TAP WATER CAN CONTAIN

Substance	Effects on the body.
Calcium Carbonate	Hardening of arteries, deterioration of internal organs, dementure.
Gasoline and MTBE (gasoline additive)	Cancer and Leukaemia.
Chlorine resistant parasites	Gastrointestinal illness, infections.
Chlorine and related hydrocarbons (DDT, PCB, TCE, etc)	Mutation, cancer, heart disease, senility.
Fluoride	Mottling of teeth, damaged immune system, Down's syndrome, heart problems, headaches, cataracts, eczema, diabetes, hair loss, still births, leukaemia, M.S, osteoporosis, cancer plus many more symptoms.
Recycled drugs (flushed down the toilet) – antibiotics, birth control pills, pain killers etc.	Lowering of male sperm count, immune system damage, brain damage plus many more symptoms.

Pesticides and herbicides (from agricultural runoff)	Mutation, birth defects, oxygen starvation, still births, heart and artery disease, cancer.
Lead from old pipes	Impairment of reproductive and central nervous systems, high blood pressure, damaged hearing, anaemia, kidney damage, mental retardation.
Acid rain	Multiple symptoms.
Arsenic (from agricultural pesticide runoff)	Damaged digestive tract and lungs, fatigue.
Aluminium	Degenerative brain damage.
Nitrates (from agricultural runoff and seepage from septic tanks)	Cancer and 'blue baby' syndrome.
Iron (as rust)	Not dangerous.
Radioactivity (from atomic power-military-medical pollution)	Birth defects, mutations, cancer.
Mercury	Loss of muscle control, kidney disease, brain damage.

ALTERNATIVES TO TAP WATER

Water type	Benefits	Drawbacks
Mineral water	Can taste good, contains some beneficial minerals, can contain biological energy (prana/chi).	Often contains harmful chemicals and inorganic, indigestible minerals.

Spring water	Convenient, can be very pure due to intensive purification techniques.	Often contains harmful chemicals and inorganic, indigestible minerals.
Carbon block filters (installed under the sink)	Kills bacteria, provides water on demand, use no electricity, easy to install.	Can not remove inorganic chemicals.
Charcoal filtered (Britta jug etc)	Cheapest and quickest option.	As above, some bacteria can still be present in filtered water, the filter can become a breeding ground for bacteria if not kept clean, it is sometimes hard to know exactly when a filter needs replacing.
Reverse osmosis water	Doesn't use electricity, produces a very pure water.	Uses 6 times more water than it produces, plumber installation required, replacement membranes costly, cannot remove all toxins.
Distilled water	100% pure. Cleanses and heals the body.	Basic home distillers are fairly expensive, also consume use a lot of electricity and take time to distil the water.

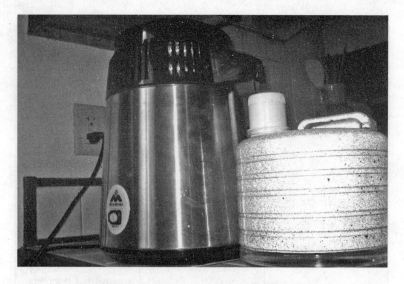

Fig. 2.2 A standard home water distiller/carbon
filter costs around £150

SOME BENEFITS OF REGULAR WATER INTAKE

> Anti aging
> Cleans the blood
> Raises energy levels
> Promotes a healthy skin
> Helps to overcome disease
> Helps to keep the joints supple
> Boosts immunity
> Promotes sharper mental capacities
> Brings homeostasis to the body's cooling and heating processes

> Helps to reduce stress, anxiety and depression
> Counters addictive tendencies
> Gives lustre and shine to the eyes
> Breaks down and energies food ready for bodily assimilation
> Effectively transports all substances within the body
> Prevents DNA damage and helps repair damaged DNA

WATER FACTS

> The idea of adding fluoride to America's tap water was first proposed in 1939 by Dr. Gerald Cox or the Mellon Institute, a research organisation that is funded by the Mellon family, owners of the Alcoa Aluminium. Fluoride is a waste product of the aluminium industry and it was claimed that it would reduce the incidence of tooth cavities.

> The best method for purifying water is a system that distils water and then carbon filters it.

> Osteoporosis affects 20 million and kills 300,000 Americans yearly. This condition is caused primarily by low quality, toxic water.

> There is approximately 326 million cubic miles of water on (and in) planet Earth.

> Water is indestructible.

> When you take a drug with a glass of water to swallow it, the water is often doing you more good than the medication.

> Ulcers are primarily caused by dehydration.

> A mere 2% drop in body water can trigger fuzzy short-term memory, trouble with basic maths and difficulty regarding focusing on the computer screen or on a printed page.

> Even mild dehydration will slow down one's metabolism as much as 3%.

Dehydration symptoms

According to Dr. Batmanghelidj's research, dehydration symptoms can fall under three broad headings:

> ➢ Perceptive feelings
> ➢ Drought management programs
> ➢ Emergency indications of local dehydration

Perceptive feelings	Drought management programs	Emergency indications of local dehydration
Tiredness	Asthma	Heartburn
Flushed face	Allergies	Dyseptic pain
Irritability	Hypertension/High blood pressure	Angina pain
Anxiousness	Type 2 diabetes	Lower back pain
Dejectedness	Constipation	Rheumatoid joint pain
Depression	Autoimmune diseases	Migraines
Heavy headedness		Colitis pain

Disturbed sleep		Fibromyalgia pains
Anger		Morning sickness during pregnancy
Impatience		Bulimia
Diminished attention span		
Shortness of breath		
Cravings for manufactured beverages		
Dreaming of water		

Perceptive feelings of dehydration

FEELING TIRED WITHOUT A PLAUSIBLE REASON

Water is integral to energy creation in the body because food cannot give energy without first being hydrolysed. And it is the hydroelectricity that fuels the energy for our neurotransmission. Due to this fact the nerve pathways and its connections to muscles and joints need to be correctly hydrated so the electricity in the body can flow easily.

FEELING FLUSHED

The brain is the most important organ of the body and is said to have up to 86% water content. If the brain becomes even marginally dehydrated, irreversible brain damage can occur, so the intelligence of the body will take attempt to avoid this by dilating the blood vessels that reach the brain.

IRRITABILITY

I've noticed in my own life that if I drink some coffee and don't follow it with plenty of water to compensate I become irritable. Dr.

Batmangelidj says that this irritability is a 'cop out' process whereby the person does not engage in brain-energy-consuming involvement beyond that particular moment.

ANXIOUSNESS

Anxiousness is a simple way that the bodily intelligence communicates its own anxiety at being dehydrated directly to the personality. In my own experience I've given clearly anxious patients a large glass of water and observed them calm down in less than a minute.

FEELING DEJECTED

Amino acids are the capital assets of the body and during dehydration these amino acids are constantly being depleted. Without a suitable amount of amino acids, the body simply cannot perform the functions it was designed to do and this inadequacy is communicated as feelings of dejection.

DEPRESSION

As the years of unintentional chronic dehydration go by, the drought in the body can become very serious. Our metabolism creates a large residue of toxic waste and ever more anti-oxidants need to be created to help to cope up with this condition. The amino acids tryptophan and tyrosine are secreted in the liver as anti-oxidants which help to clean up the toxicity.

The tryptophan is needed for the brain to produce serotonin, melatonin, tryptamine and indolamine. These elements are key neurotransmitters that balance and integrate body functions. And the depletion of these elements leads to our depression.

The Tyrosine is used by the brain to create adrenaline, noradrenaline and dopamine. These elements have been called the 'go getter' neurotransmitters whose depletion will ground the personality with inactivity and a sorrowful feeling.

HEAVY HEADEDNESS

This is an indication that the brain is commanding an increased flow of blood circulation for its hydration needs. The brain cells create waste during metabolism and without adequate hydration, these acidic toxins can build up that eventually lead to migraines.

ANGER

Anger is a more expressive way of showing our irritability.

DIMINISHED ATTENTION SPAN

Focussing the attention takes energy. The more hydrated the brain; the more energy it can manufacture. So in case the brain does not have adequate energy supply from water (hydro-electric energy) a process of disengagement will occur which can result in losing attention and possibly makes us becoming impatient.

CRAVINGS FOR MANUFACTURED BEVERAGES

Drinks such as tea, coffee and soda are diuretic in nature and only serve to further dehydrate the body, yet due to conditioning, many of us reflexively reach out for these toxic drinks when feeling dehydrated.

Drought management programs

ASTHMA

High levels of histamine are created in the body as a drought management mechanism to promote drinking water and ration the water that is already available. In many cases related to asthma, there is heightened histamine content in the tissues of the lungs. There are tiny air sacks in the lungs are called alveoli and it is through these miniscule holes that water evaporates through the lungs. In a simple manoeuvre, histamine and its subordinates constrict the alveoli and this causes asthma symptoms.

ALLERGIES

In addition to its water regulatory function, histamine also acts as an agent to defend the body against harmful bacteria and foreign materials. In a hydrated body, these histamic processes will be silent and unexaggerated, however in a dehydrated body it will give rise to exaggerated responses.

HYPERTENSION/HIGH BLOOD PRESSURE

In a condition when the fluid volume in the blood decreases due to dehydration, the vessels need to reduce their aperture (contract) in order to prevent the occurrence 'gas locks', this creates high blood pressure. Treating hypertension with diuretics makes no sense whatsoever; water is the ultimate natural diuretic.

TYPE 2 DIABETES

An end result of chronic water shortage in the body is when the serotonergic neurotransmitter system is affected. It has been shown that in a diabetic brain, serotonin levels are diminished and thus it is forced to raise its glucose levels to adequately power the brain and its various functions. Insulin imports glucose to the brain cells yet the hydroelectric creation of energy in the diabetic brain is preferential to energy derived from glucose (sugar).

CONSTIPATION

When the body is in need of extra water, the walls of the colon involuntarily contract in order to extract moisture from the compacted faecal matter that is stored there. Then this faecal-extracted moisture is reintroduced into the body via the lining membranes of the colon walls. Constipation is caused by the body holding on to the faecal matter longer than normal in order to allow the re-absorption of the water content of the waste matter.

AUTOIMMUNE DISEASES

After speaking with dozens of Multiple Sclerosis patients, I noticed that every single one of them was chronically dehydrated.

In extreme cases, persistent cellular dehydration will result in a number of disruptive health conditions that have been labelled as different diseases depending on the specialty of the 'medical specialist' who first labels the problem. In the early stages, amino acids become depleted as antioxidants, and due to the fact the body is not creating enough urine to detoxify the body sufficiently against the waste of metabolism. A knock-on effect of this amino acid depletion also results in the subsequent depletion of neurotransmitters such as serotonin, typtamine, melatonin and indolamine (made from the amino acid tryptophan) or adrenaline, noradrenalline and dopamine (that are made up from the amino acid tryptophan).

Instead of recognising conditions such as Multiple Sclerosis, Muscular Dystrophy, Amyotrophic Lateral Ssclerosis (Lou Gehrig's disease), Parkinson's disease and Alzheimer's disease as deficiency disorders, the medical profession simply label them as 'diseases of unknown cause'. And instead of correcting the dehydration and its metabolic complications, patients are given toxic medications.

Emergency indications of local dehydration

HEARTBURN & DYSPEPTIC PAIN

Gastritis, duodenitis, heart burn, and colitis are caused by excess acidity in the stomach which the dehydrated body cannot adequately defend itself against. Water washes the mucous that lines the stomach thus removing its salt deposits. When water is lacking, the mucous cannot effectively neutralise the stomach acid.

ANGINA PAIN

Angina is a signal of dehydration in the lung/heart area. The blood of a dehydrated person is concentrated and the heart has to work harder to pump it around the body. This leads to an unnerving tight chest sensation.

LOWER BACK PAIN

Cartilage is the substance that prevents bones from sheering together in joints and is made up primarily of water and salt. The lower part of the spine carries a proportionally high percentage of the body's weight and thus is one of the first areas to suffer from dehydration-caused joint pain. It is important for water to be able to enter the spaces between the vertebral discs for circulatory purposes. In a dehydrated state, the discs can press on local nerves giving a painful 'twinge' or a steady, dull pain throughout the day.

RHEUMATOID JOINT PAIN

About eight million people in the UK are said to suffer from some kind of arthritic pain with an extimated $16 million spent annually in the US on back pain treatment alone.

Joint pain often occurs because there is not enough water to wash out the local acidity and toxic substances. Where the pain is felt is where the localised drought has settled.

MIGRAINES

Blood vessels leading from the heart to the brain will dilate when the body is dehydrated to allow extra blood to reach the brain, especially during warm nights under the bed covers. These same arteries (carotid arteries) lead to the scalp and the face as well, which is why some headaches begin with pulsating arteries around the temples.

Migraine headaches can be extremely painful and incapacitating. Medical doctors will often tell patients that there is no cure for headaches and instead they will prescribe painkillers (such as aspirin), vasoconstrictors and nausea tablets to suppress the symptoms. In some cases even calcium channel blockers are used as a so-called 'preventative' yet one of their many side effects is a headache.

COLITIS PAIN

This refers to pain in the lower left hand side of the abdomen. For the final products of food digestion to pass through the intestinal tract, the lubricating property of water is essential. Peristaltic activity in the intestines controls the passage of food and in a dehydrated body, normal peristalsis is reduced to a tighter contraction to extract moisture from the solid matter.

WaterCure is gaining worldwide approval

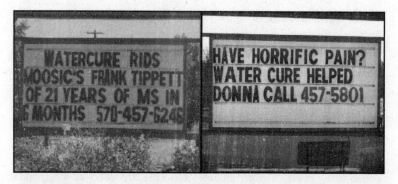

Bob Butts in the US is an excellent example of a 'regular guy' spreading core information about the WaterCure because he feels a moral obligation to do so. He spends much of his spare time and money on advertising initiatives to spread Dr. Batmanghelidj's message: 'You are not sick, you are thirsty'.

His website contains an impressive collection of testimonials from people who have overcome a wide range of illnesses using water and salt. He also has links to some fascinating TV appearances made by Dr. Batmanghelidj and himself promoting the WaterCure.

Bob's campaign includes adverts in the Citizens Voice Newspaper which clearly mention that even critical conditions like advanced cancer have responded to the Water Cure Treatment.

It is not possible to capitalise on the WaterCure in the same way that it is with medications and remedies due to its highly simple nature; yet the formula of water and salt is spreading through the world via word of mouth, small-scale local promotion and via Dr. Batmanghelidj's books, audio and video cassettes. His various books are available from larger stores and from the Internet. These books are written in a way that both the layman and professional medical practitioner can clearly understand the pivotal role of unintentional dehydration in disease.

Water Q&A

Can I drink too much water?

Technically yes, however up to as much as four or five litres per day should not cause any adverse effects. Always take the correct amount of salt in comparison to how much water you are drinking and build up to the desired intake steadily over a few weeks, if you've been chronically dehydrated for a long time.

I drink lots of tea and coffee each day, does this count as water?

No, it doesn't, as the dehydrating effects of caffeine (especially coffee) necessitate drinking more water afterwards to compensate. Drinking at least as much water again after tea and double the amount again after coffee is a recommended guideline.

I drink lots of beer, which is mainly water, does that count?

As above.

I don't like drinking water, what should I do?

If you don't enjoy drinking pure water then something must be wrong. Learn to enjoy water by treating it as the essential life-giving elixir that it is. Make herbal tea if you prefer and try to avoid drinking unfiltered tap water if possible.

I don't want to have to go to the toilet all the time.

If you don't drink enough water, you'll pay the price of sickness and premature death. You choose! Having to urinate every few hours is not a reason to starve your body of water.

I don't seem to be able to hold the water I drink inside for long, is there anything I can do about this?

Yes, take the salt remedy every day. You probably need to increase the electrolytes in your blood, which can be achieved by taking real salt every day. Also do some exercises every day, especially 'sit-up' style ones to strengthen the bladder.

In the summer I find it easy to drink lots of water but in the winter I don't feel like it due to the cold weather. How do you manage to keep hydrated during the cold months?

I have a 1.5 litre thermos flask, which I fill with boiling water twice a day. There is always a pint glass and various herbal tea bags close to hand and I just keep filling up the glass with hot water when necessary. I try to avoid drinking water that is at room temperature but that doesn't stop me taking a water bottle with me when I leave the house for a few hours. If I drink cool water I make sure to swill it around my mouth first to warm it up.

I've been drinking tap water and want to change but I don't have much spare cash.

For anyone who can possibly afford it, I would suggest purchasing a water distiller, however if this is not possible or convenient, I recommend finding a suitable bottled water or getting a water filter to go by the sink (prices start at about £18).

I have kidney problems and my doctor told me to avoid salt. Is the WaterCure correct for me?

If your kidneys are not working well, then don't follow this program without first seeking competent health advice. If you still want to try it on your own, drink one full glass of water and wait until you go to the bathroom. Then drink another glass. When your kidneys come up to speed (input matches output), then start the salt slowly to make sure your kidneys are working ok.

How can I find out more about my local tap water?

Look up your local water board and ask them to send you the information that you require. If you can smell chemicals when you turn the tap on, you can be sure the water is dangerous to drink.

I'm trying to drink more water but keep forgetting.

Plan ahead and make it easy for yourself. You could leave bottles of water in rooms where you spend most of your time (eg: one in the living room, one in the bedroom, one at work etc). Also you could fill up a large pot/flask/caffetiere with herbal tea and have it by you to drink at regular intervals. Make a commitment to take a drink each and every time you get the thought to drink water.

A few years ago, I 'initiated' a three-year-old friend into the 'mystery of crystal salt' by giving him a rock of it and telling him it was the 'magic salt licker'. Every time God tells him to lick the rock, he must lick the rock. When he licks the rock, it will make him a little bit thirsty, so he must drink some water...then he will become strong like daddy! It was charming to watch him playing with his brother, then as if a 'force from the outside' had taken hold of him, he would stop what he was doing, lick the rock and have a swig of water from his magic bottle, then carry on playing happily.

When to drink water

Whilst medical students are taught that dry mouth is the first sign of dehydration, Dr. Batmanghelidj points out that actually it is one of the last. He makes his point clearly when he says 'waiting to get thirsty is waiting to die prematurely of chronic, unintentional dehydration.' Upon awakening, it is important to drink plenty of water because as the body sleeps, it loses water through processes such as sweating and evaporation through exhalation. So, it is also wise to drink water before going to bed at night, warm water with a pinch of salt works wonderfully at both times – in the morning, it gives the body a 'shot' of up to 85 minerals in an easily digested, liquid form and in the evening, the salt acts as a mild hypnotic, aiding easy sleep.

Water should also be drunk regularly throughout the day, so as to keep saline and hydration levels balanced at all times. It is advisable to carry a bottle of water when away from the vicinity of a tap. Rather than waiting until your body is showing signs of advanced dehydration (such as a dry mouth, dizziness and nausea), aim to proactively keep dehydration at bay. After starting the WaterCure, the body will gradually begin to recognise even the slightest fall in hydration levels and will send a signal to the brain – not a 'crisis call' but rather a gentle whisper – 'hey, friend…take a swig from the bottle…it's good for you.' When you receive this message, don't postpone drinking until later, it is the subconscious mind talking to your personality and the advice is good, so there's only one loser in the 'waiting to get thirsty' game; and it is you!

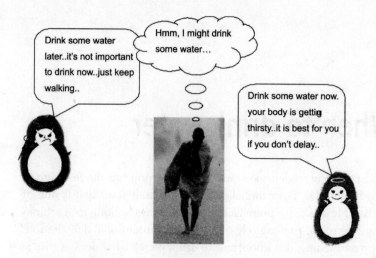

Drinking a glass of water half an hour before eating a meal will provide the body with the hydration it requires to properly assimilate the food via the action of hydrolysis. It is best to avoid drinking much water for two hours after eating a meal as the water will dilute the digestive acids and creates a 'pool' of food and water in the stomach. Whilst drinking water should be a regular part of daily life, always keep the following diagram in mind as a general guideline.

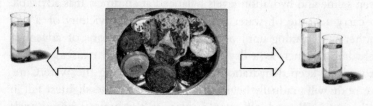

30 minutes before   **2 hours after**

Misinforming the public about hydration

The vested interest lobby groups and bogus non-governmental organisations incessantly expose us to outrageous pseudo-science in order to sell us their dubious products and services. A good example of this is how the tea industry pays doctors to say nice things about tea, even if that means lying.

TEA 'HEALTHIER' DRINK THAN WATER

Thursday, 24 August 2006

'Drinking three or more cups of tea a day is as good for you as drinking plenty of water and may even have extra health benefits', say researchers.

The work in the European Journal of Clinical Nutrition dispels the common belief that tea dehydrates.

Tea not only rehydrates as well as water does, but it can also protect you against heart disease and some cancers, UK nutritionists found.

The experts believe flavonoids, the key ingredient in tea that promotes health.

Healthy cuppa

These polyphenol antioxidants are found in many foods and plants, including tea leaves, and have been shown to help prevent cell damage.

Tea replaces fluids and contains antioxidants so its got two things going for it.

Public health nutritionist Dr Carrie Ruxton, and his colleagues at Kings College London, looked at published studies on the health effects of tea consumption.

They found clear evidence that drinking three to four cups of tea a day can cut the chances of having a heart attack.

Some studies also suggested that tea consumption protected against cancer, although this effect was less clear-cut.

Other health benefits seen included protection against tooth plaque and potentially tooth decay, plus bone strengthening.

Dr Ruxton said: 'Drinking tea is actually better for you than drinking water. Water is essentially replacing fluid. Tea replaces fluids and contains antioxidants so it's got two things going for it.'

Rehydrating

She said it was an urban myth that tea is dehydrating.

'Studies on caffeine have found very high doses dehydrate and everyone assumes that caffeine-containing beverages dehydrate. But even if you had a really, really strong cup of tea or coffee, which is quite hard to make, you would still have a net gain of fluid.'

'Also, a cup of tea contains fluoride, which is good for the teeth,' she added.

There was no evidence that tea consumption was harmful to

health. However, research suggests that tea can impair the body's ability to absorb iron from food, meaning people at risk of anaemia should avoid drinking tea around mealtimes.

'Tea is not dehydrating. It is a healthy drink'.? Claire Williamson of the British Nutrition Foundation. Dr Ruxton's team found average tea consumption was just under three cups per day. She said the increasing popularity of soft drinks meant many people were not drinking as much tea as before.

'Tea drinking is most common in older people, the 40 plus age range. In older people, tea sometimes made up about 70% of fluid intake, so it is a really important contributor,' she said. Claire Williamson of the British Nutrition Foundation said: 'Studies in the laboratory have shown potential health benefits.'

'The evidence in humans is not as strong and more studies need to be done. But there are definite potential health benefits from the polyphenols in terms of reducing the risk of diseases such as heart disease and cancers.'

'In terms of fluid intake, we recommend 1.5-2 litres per day and that can include tea. Tea is not dehydrating. It is a healthy drink.'

The Tea Council provided funding for the work. Dr Ruxton stressed that the work was independent.

Upon further investigation, Dr Carrie Ruxton seems to be the only visible member of a company called 'Nutrition-Communications'.

In her biography, it states that she has 'particular skill with hostile/sceptical audiences', is a 'practitioner of persuasion, logic & perseverance', has a 'diplomatic approach to crisis management' and is 'committed to evidence-based argument'. I'll bet she is! Committed to her own bogus 'evidence' and an expert at changing people's minds and dealing people who are angry with the lies of corporate 'healthcare' interests, which of course are deeply enmeshed with the UK government and many other governments worldwide.

I had to laugh when I read how Nutrition Communications can benefit customers:

'When promoting messages to the media, consumers, healthcare professionals or to opinion-leaders, companies benefit enormously from an independent voice. Carrie Ruxton and her team offer the ideal combination of professional credibility and flexible communications skills.

The fast pace of the communication environment requires consultants who can handle a range of situations. Having built up experience over a number of years and with many different clients, Nutrition Communications staff require little supervision and can respond to a short brief and tight deadlines.

'Fees are from £550 per day, with discounts for blocks of 10 or more days, for long-term projects or the public sector.'

So basically, for a few thousand pounds she'll make an unhealthy product sound healthy so as to deceive the general public.

'The Nutritional Communications' links to a site claims that table salt is just as good as 'polish salt'; another treacherous and dangerous lie and another site which makes E-numbers and sweeteners such as Aspartame sound safe.

One week around the end of May in the UK the various newspapers all decided to trumpet the 'discovery' that actually we don't need to drink much water to be healthy. I decided to collect the various articles and stick them on a large sheet of cardboard, so I could show people how the propaganda machine works. From the Sun to the Times to the Metro to the Independent; all the journalists were singing from the same song sheet.

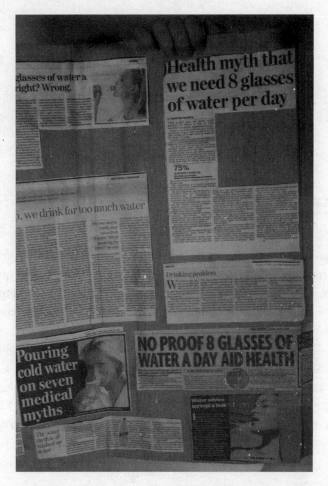

Fig. 2.3 Newspaper inscripts clearing myths related to water

I need to say no more than this; next time you notice some so-called expert intoning on the BBC (or any other mass media channel) that black is white and white is black, recognize that you may be being lied to.

Testimonies

'I never really thought about drinking water regularly until a friend said my skin was looking dry. I started drinking a pint of mild herbal tea regularly and very quickly noticed many benefits including a much softer and healthier skin, brighter eyes and an end to my periodic headaches. Basically, I feel much younger and healthier.'

- James, London

'In 2 minutes a bad headache was relieved 95% by drinking a glass of warm salt water followed by a glass of regular water. I have suffered from headaches for many years and never thought to drink more water before.'

- Patricia, London

'I have Multiple Sclerosis. I have been using the WaterCure about a month now. All I can say is that I have discovered a miracle. Prior to starting to use this simple plan, I had chronic muscle spasms and that were very, very, very painful. I have tried a number of things including physical therapy, muscle stimulators, pain medication and etc. All just gave temporary relief and only hurt my pocketbook. I believe my eyesight and balance have improved and I know my pain and fatigue have been alleviated 95%!

I would like to thank Dr. B. from the bottom of my heart for discovering and sharing this free medicine! I have been able to stop all RX medication! Yeah!'

- Jackie Saxton

'I have been suffering with rheumatoid arthritis pain. The pain in my joints was so severe, I could hardly walk. I had spent so much time, energy and now most of the money I had saved, and still I was in pain. I had read about the body's cries for water some time ago, and I remembered it was very good, but until recently when a friend suggested that I read your book on RA and back pain, did I remember how potent the water cure could be. I started having most of the joint problems after I moved to the high desert. I didn't drink much water before I moved, and in the last two years, I have not increased my intake of water. Afterwards I read the book, I started drinking water in the AM, two glasses, a half hour before a meal, then more water two hours after. I find I have usually had problems in drinking water, but now, the more I drink, the more I want, and I am recognizing my so called hunger as thirst. For the first time in 2 years, I am once again able to walk over a mile at a time. I am experiencing less and less pain and swelling in my ankles, knees, wrists, and other joints. I am 30 lbs overweight, and hope that being able to walk and move will help this situation as well.'

- Rebecca Clemons

'Even though I don't have any health complaints, I still drink a small cup of hot salt water each morning as it helps to wake me up and get bolstered for the day.'

- Graham, London

'I have drunk loads of water each day for most of my life (around five litres each day), I just love it. Then I was told about how important the salt is and since I've started adding real salt (as opposed to the table salt) to my food and mixing it with water sometimes and my previous problems (coughs, colds, runny nose, sore throat etc) have gone and not come back. I also have a lot more energy.'

- Susan, Southampton

'I was absolutely shocked when I read the chapters on water and salt in the Five Point Plan. I always assumed that salt intake was the cause of high blood pressure because that's what the doctors always seem to be saying here in the UK. I have since learned that there is a vast difference between 'table' salt and 'real salt'. Applying the simple WaterCure formula to my life has made me feel lighter, fitter and my complexion has improved tremendously.'

Jennifer, London

Summary

I believe that the first two things to be checked while ascertaining the health of a patient are the water and salt balance. Often ignored completely by medical doctors and relegated to nothing more than an afterthought by naturopaths and homeopaths ('...oh, and remember to drink enough water as well.'), the role of unintentional chronic dehydration in disease is of pivotal, undeniable and obvious importance. It is not just a question of drinking lots of water because unless real salt is obtained in the correct amounts each day, mineral deficiency and its myriad related complications will eventually manifest.

SALT

'Ye are the salt of the earth: but if the salt have lost his savour, wherewith shall it be salted? It is thenceforth good for nothing, but to be cast out, and to be trodden under foot of men.'

- Bible, New Testament, Matthew 5:13

Introduction

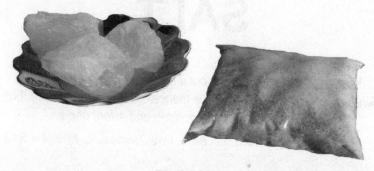

Fig. 3.1 Salt

Is salt good for us? Depending on the type of salt we are talking about, the answer can be either yes or no. In a nutshell, refined/table salt only contains sodium chloride plus a few harmful chemicals, whereas real salt (pure sea salt or rock salt) is essential for a healthy life.

The real salts are necessary to live healthily because they contain 85+ vital minerals, trace minerals, elements and organic compounds that are essential to keep the body in good working order. Don't buy into the 'salt is dangerous' model as salt deficiency is a major cause of disease in the modern world. If you are avoiding salt or using refined table salt, you are inviting serious trouble into your life. It is widely believed that the ingredients that real salts contain are necessary for all creatures because they had to be present in the ocean-water lagoon where single cell organisms developed on Earth around a billion years ago.

Both sea salt and rock salt were well known to the ancient Greeks who used it for medical purposes. The healing methods of Hippocrates (460 BC) especially made frequent use of salt. Salt-based folk remedies can be highly effective and should definitely be used more in modern life instead of relying on expensive and largely ineffectual chemical alternatives. Examples of such remedies include drinking a mixture of two-thirds cow's milk and one-third salt-water in the mornings and on an empty stomach. This remedy was recommended as a cure for diseases of the spleen and a mixture of salt and honey was applied topically to clean bad ulcers. Salt-water was used externally against infected wounds and skin diseases.

A closer look at salt

The table salt is basically only sodium chloride plus a few harmful chemicals; all of the other beneficial elements have been removed. Most of the salt available in the supermarkets is not suitable, sometimes even if it says 'sea salt' on the label. In the UK for instance any salt can be labelled 'sea salt' if it has been obtained from the sea, irrespective of the refinement processes that may have taken place afterwards. Ideally look for a moist salt or a salt in rock/crystal form, which are widely available from health stores and some of the better supermarkets. Regular table salt that can be easily poured through a saltshaker has been stripped of its companion elements and contains additives such as aluminium silicate to keep it powdery and porous.

Aluminium is a very toxic element in our nervous system and is implicated as one of the primary causes of Alzheimer's disease. Regular table salt has been harvested mechanically from dirt or concrete basins, put through intensive and degrading artificial processes heated under extreme temperatures of up to 1200 degrees F to crack its molecular structure and robbed of its essential minerals that are essential to our physiology. In addition to all this, harmful chemicals have been added to mask all the impurities that it has, such

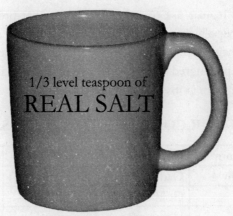

1/3 level teaspoon of
REAL SALT

Fig. 3.2 Real Salt

as free flowing agents, inorganic iodine and bleaching agents. The salt that we take must be untreated, unheated and unrefined to be truly effective as a life enhancing, healing elixir.

In his comprehensive book 'Salt Deficiency', Martin Lara recommends drinking a cup of hot water with a third to one-half a level teaspoon of sea-salt upon awakening and before bed each night. Such a simple elixir can dramatically help with many conditions, such as:

• Pneumonia	• Constipation	• Vomiting
• Diarrhoea	• BloatingColitis	• Bronchitis
• Stomach pain	• Stomach viruses	• Acid indigestion
• Common colds	• Heart disease	• Low immunity
• Influenza	• Sore throat	• Morning sickness
• 'Strep' throat	• Mucus/phlegm	• Tuberculosis
• Migraine headaches	• Haemorrhoids	• Yeast infection
• Colon cancer	• Psoriasis	• Acne

With regular use of salt it is unlikely that problems will arise again, especially if it is used coupled with a healthy diet and lifestyle. The hot, salt water is a wonderfully effective elixir because it contains the elemental ingredients our body requires to function properly and also make correct use of the water we drink.

THE MAJOR COMPONENTS OF SEA SALT

Aluminium	Flourine	Neodymium	Silicon
Antimony	Gadolinium	Nickel	Silver
Arsenic	Gold	Niobium	Strontium
Barium	Hafnium	Nitrogen	Tantalum
Beryllium	Holmium	Osmium	Terbium
Bismuth	Indium	Palladium	Thallium
Boron	Iodine	Phosphorus	Thorium
Bromine	Iridium	Platinum	Thulium
Cadmium	Iron	Potassium	Tin
Carbon	Lanthanum	Praseodymium	Titanium
Caesium	Lead	Rhenium	Tungsten
Chromium	Lithium	Rhodium	Uranium
Cobalt	Lutetium	Rubidium	Vanadium
Copper	Magnesium	Ruthenium	Ytterbium
Dysprosium	Manganese	Samarium	Yttrium
Erbium	Mercury	Scandium	Zinc
Europium	Molybdenum	Selenium	Zirconium

Some benefits of real Salt

> Maintains proper hydration

> Boosts the immune system

> Helps the body to digest foods properly

> Keeps the body well hydrated

> Prevents constipation

> Aids communication between the brain, cells and bacteria

> Repairs wounds and regenerates cells

> Creates an internal environment that is unfavourable to the malignant micro-organisms

> Prevents premature aging and disease

> Maintains the conductivity that the nervous system requires to send and receive the electrical impulses needed to communicate with all the organs, muscles and glands in the body

> Boosts the efficiency of all the white blood cells

> Produces a type of hydrochloric acid that can offer protection from many diseases that infect the intestines

- ➤ Increases the production of saliva, a potent antiseptic and healing secretion
- ➤ Maintains control of all the malignant and benign micro-organisms in our intestines, which digest and restructure the food needed for sustenance
- ➤ Regulates blood pressure
- ➤ Clears the lungs of mucus and sticky phlegm, particularly in asthma and cystic fibrosis
- ➤ Prevents muscle cramps
- ➤ Makes firm bone structure
- ➤ Regulates sleep
- ➤ Maintains sexuality and libido
- ➤ Prevents varicose veins

Interesting Salt facts

- ➤ Given the health differences between pure salt and refined salt, we might expect that doctors would know the difference, yet in most cases they don't

- ➤ If the salt collects on the bottom of the glass after stirring, it has been processed. Natural salt always dissolves quite easily. Salt that will not dissolve in water cannot dissolve in your body, leading to several diseases

- ➤ Our pets also suffer from salt deficiency because most pet food contains excessive amounts of refined salt. Farmers place rock salt-blocks on their pasture so that their livestock and all other animals can lick those blocks it as much as they like. Animals always benefit from such procedures. They drink more water when a salt-lick is present as well

- ➤ Keep a bottle of salt water handy (approximately 1/3 of a level teaspoon per pint of water) and leave out two bowls for your pet at home, one containing normal water and the other containing the salt water. The pet can then benefit from all that the salt offers without getting dehydrated

> If every particle of salt were taken from our body, we would live for about 48 hours.

> Tears are salty and so is blood. Salt bathes a body's tissues. A solution of salt water substituted for blood lost will keep a human or animal alive for hours

> In Asia Minor, stone axes were found in salt quarries indicating that salt was used by those primitive people during the Neolithic period

> Tribal kings and priests of ancient Mexico, Peru, Egypt, Babylon and other civilisations seized control of salt wherever it was found. By regulating it, they held the power of life and death over their subjects. They could demand anything they desired – for a pinch of salt

> Homer, who lived about 550 B.C. called salt 'divine'. Plato said salt was 'dear to the gods'

> One of the greatest military roads in history was built to bring salt from the salt works in Ostia, on the Tiber river, to Rome. This road is called the Via Salaria and is still in use today

> Romans were paid in part with salt coins that were called 'solarium' from which came the English word 'salary'

> Mahatma Gandhi's Salt March brought about the freedom of India from British colonial rule and the tyranny of salt taxation

> Since electrolysed water contains sea/rock salt it promotes regular bowel movements. Once bowel regularity is achieved the cause of bad breath, for instance, vanishes

Q&A

Is it really as simple as you say?

Not always, but usually it is. In many cases illness vanishes very quickly after intake of sea salt and water is increased. The most powerful truths are always simple; try for yourself and see.

I keep forgetting to take the salt remedy, any tips?

Ways to help you remember to take salt include keeping small bags of salt in places where you spend most of your time and taking a pinch when you think to, being more regimented about when you take your salt remedy (e.g. every morning/evening at the same time each day), making up a salt/water solution in a bottle and keeping it in a place where you will see it every day.

Where can I get good rock/crystal/sea salt?

Health food shops, decent supermarkets, markets, butchers, Internet etc.

Can taking the salt remedy have adverse effects?

Only if the body is dehydrated so as ever, make sure you drink plenty of water through the day. If too much salt is taken and not enough water, high blood pressure, acidity and other problems will result. People with weak kidneys should exercise caution (see the Water chapter: Q&A).

If real salt can save us and table salt can kills us, how come we don't learn about it at school, college or even medical college?

According to Dr. Batmanghelidj, the information about water and salt is fraudulently and methodologically suppressed by the upper levels of the pharmaceutical 'powers that be'. Students and doctors are usually unaware of the difference between real and duplicate salt because the courses they study deliberately don't cover the difference. Why? If you can control the water and salt of a country/civilisation you can control the population's health and ultimately their lives. Gandhi's Salt March comes to mind as a slightly different example of how invaders took control of the salt in order to control the population. The Raj wanted to control the tax on the salt and Gandhi defeated their chicanery; yet each year when I return to India I see more and more toxic 'free-flow' and 'iodized' salt on the restaurant tables and in the shops. The colonialists may have been ousted but it would appear that certain 'forces of evil' are poisoning India's water and salt like they are in many other parts of the world.

Himalayan crystal salt

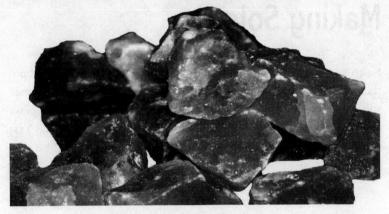

Fig. 3.3 Himalayan Crystal Salt

The himalayan crystal salt contains all the elements of which the human body is comprised of. From the periodic table of elements, we are familiar with 94 natural elements (stable as well as unstable). Apart from the so-called inert gases, these elements can be found in crystal salt. Hence, crystal salt contains all natural minerals and trace elements that are found in the human body. Thanks in part to a substantial global marketing campaign from companies selling products such as 'Original Himalayan Crystal Salt', people are starting to use high quality salt and turn their backs on the grossly inferior, toxic-to-the-body table salt.

Making Sole

Keep adding salt to a glass of water untill you'll get to a point where the water becomes saturated with salt. When the water becomes super-saturated the crystal rock will sit on the bottom of the glass without dissolving. This is what salt sole (pronounced 'so-lay') is; super-saturated salty water.

Step 1

Place 1 inch of Himalayan crystal salt stones in a glass jar, preferably one with a lid. Add 2 to 3 inches of good quality water above the stones, completely covering the crystals with water. Let it sit overnight.

Step 2

If all the salt crystals have dissolved, add a few more salt crystals to the water. The sole is ready when the water becomes fully saturated with salt and cannot hold any more. The salt will no longer dissolve at this stage. There should always be salt crystals in the jar. As you use up the sole, after some time, add more water and more salt until the water is again saturated. Remember, there should always be undissolved salt crystals on the bottom of the jar. This is your visual proof that the water is super-saturated with salt.

Step 3

Each morning, before eating or drinking anything, add one teaspoon of the sole to a glass of water and drink. Your body will receive the energetic vibration pattern of the salt and hold it for twenty four hours. Keep the container covered to prevent the water from evaporating. Otherwise, no special storage is needed. The fully saturated sole will keep indefinitely. Salt is a natural anti-bacterial and natural fungicide and therefore cannot spoil or go bad.

One teaspoon of 'Original Himalayan Crystal Salt' sole contains 478 mg of sodium (equivalent to 20% of the USDA's recommended daily allowance of 2,500 mg.) A 1% Sole solution is 1 part sole and 99 parts water.

Percentage of Solution	Amount of Crystal Salt	Amount of Water	Application
1% Sole Solution	1/2 teaspoon. (2g)	200ml	For Eyes & Nose
"	2 teaspoon. (10g)	1000ml	For Inhalation
"	1 Kilo (2.2 lbs.)	100 litre to a bath tub	For sole bathing

Amongst health enthusiasts there are sometimes discussions about which type of salt is the best. In favour of sea salt, Martin Lara states in his book 'Salt Deficiency' that sea salt is ideal for humans as it contains the perfect ratio of minerals for our health needs. Sea salt contains minerals from all the mountains and terrains on Earth (which are then washed out to sea), an event which has been happening over and over again for billions of years. These minerals get mixed together by tides and ocean currents and after all this time, and what we end up with is a salt that contains minerals that once could be found only in India, Australia, Italy, Alaska etc.

In my kitchen at home, I am pleased to say that I have a set of six presentation jars containing various different salts from around the world, from French Atlantic, to Malvern (UK), to powdered pink Himalayan crystals. I must confess that I nearly always carry a small pouch of decent salt with me when I go to restaurants as well.

The all important WaterCure formula

> Drink approximately 1/4 to 1/3 of your body weight (in stone) as litres of pure water per day. Or drink pure water (in litres.), approximately ¼ to 1/3 of your body weight, per day. Alternatively, you can drink pure water (in ounces), half of your body weight, per day, a half your body weight in pounds as ounces of water per day.

> Take just under 1/3 of a level teaspoon of real salt for every litre of water you drink. Put on food, mix in water etc.

> Tea, coffee, sodas, alcohol etc are diuretic liquids, which mean that they serve to make you more dehydrated than before you drank them.

> If you are unused to drinking enough water each day, build up to the optimum amount gradually.

> Avoid drinking water from the fridge, as cold liquid damages the digestive system.

It's so simple and so profoundly important!

I've been following the WaterCure for about eight years and can say with my hand on my heart that it is crucial for my health and well being; like I'm sure it is for other people. Why then do most people I know systematically fail to drink enough water and take the right amount of salt each day?

I know from my own experience that some of the reasons for people failing to get properly hydrated include:

➢ Laziness

➢ Addiction to sugary drinks

➢ Not wanting to go to the toilet regularly

➢ Not realising how important the water is

➢ Not liking the taste of chemicalised tap water and not quite managing to purchase a decent water-purifying device.

➢ Being misled by doctors and so called nutrition 'experts'

So, I urge all readers who are not drinking enough water to make a firm, conscious decision to treat water as the life-giving elixir it is and drink the correct amount each day with the correct amount of real salt.

Hot water/salt based elixirs

ELIXIR 1: HOT MOLASSES

Ingredients:

> ➤ 1 pint of hot water
> ➤ Pinch of sea/crystal salt
> ➤ 1-2 tablespoons of organic apple cider vinegar
> ➤ 1 tablespoon of organic blackstrap molasses

The nutritional content of the above drink cannot be over-stated. This drink is an ideal way to quickly, economically and simply obtain large doses of important vitamins and minerals in a way that the body can instantly make use of.

ELIXIR 2: CAYENNE WARMER

Ingredients:

> ➤ 1 Pint of hot water
> ➤ Pinch of sea/crystal salt
> ➤ 1/3 level teaspoon of organic cayenne pepper
> ➤ Juice of 1 organic lemon

> Add honey or molasses if desired

ELIXIR 3: HOT LEMON GINGER ENERGISER

Ingredients:

> 1 Pint of hot water
> Pinch of sea/crystal salt
> A few thin slices of organic ginger root (boil in water for 5 minutes)
> Juice of 1 organic lemon
> Add honey or molasses if desired

Summary

'Real salts' contain up to eighty five life giving minerals and are an integral part of our blood. Without it water cannot get into the cells of the body. This results in unintentional chronic dehydration and its many related complications.

URINE

'He, who takes Shivambu (urine) daily...acquires divine accomplishments quickly. Freed from all ailments, and possessing a body comparable to that of Shiva Himself, he disports himself like the gods in the Universe for an eternity.'

- Shiva speaks to Parvati, Damar Sutra

Introduction

Would you believe me if I told you that our number one health elixir is completely free and available to all people without any need for any marketing or distribution? How about if I told you that billions of litres of this universal medicine were literally flushed down the toilet each and every day, disregarded as waste? The healing substance is urine and when the population finally awaken to its truly extraordinary properties, disease may well become a thing of the past.

The urine is not a waste product as we have been told but rather a non-toxic biofeedback stimulator that boosts immunity by activating the immune system, thus restoring the body to an internally balanced state of health. And urine contains an impressive array of ingredients, including vitamins, minerals, proteins, amino acids and enzymes, all perfectly blended for your particular health needs.

It is not made in the intestines but rather it is made in (and by) the kidneys, making it a highly distilled form of your own blood. Re-introducing fresh urine into the body will yield instant results and allow us for the close monitoring of progress. The urine therapy is both a system of healing and diagnosis. The colour, taste and smell give away many clues as to the precise nature of your health complaint. Basically, the darker yellow the urine is, the more dehydrated you are, so it is important to drink pure water regularly, especially if you are drinking your own urine in the mornings. If the taste and smell of your urine is bad, it means your system is toxic. With the regular intake of water and a sensible diet, it tastes fine. With the administration of urine therapy you will be taking up an ancient and highly powerful practice that will lead to benefits you may not yet have imagined, so do not underestimate the body's ability to heal itself perfectly.

Despite what we have been led to believe about urine, pharmaceutical companies have made obscene profits from the sale of drugs made from urine constituents. Pergonal, a fertility drug made from human urine, earned a reported $855 million in sales in 1992, and sales ($1400 a month per patient) have increased yearly. Urokinase is marketed as a 'miracle blood clot dissolver' for unblocking coronary arteries, yet it is actually just one of the ingredients in urine! Urea, medically proven to be one of the best moisturizers in the world, is also contained in urine and is integral to cosmetic companies, who package it in expensive, glamorized creams and lotions. We can either laugh or cry as we realize that very often we are being sold our own urine back to us as 'miracles of modern science'! Make no mistake; correct information about urine is being suppressed to protect the financial interests of multi-national pharmaceutical companies and their shareholders.

A closer look at urine

'Shivambu (urine) is heavenly nectar, which is capable of destroying senility and diseases.'

- Damar tantra

In 1975, one of the founders of Miles Laboratories, Dr. A.H. Free, published his book Urinalysis in Clinical Laboratory Practice, in which he stated that urine is a sterile body compound (purer than distilled water) and that 'It is now recognized that urine contains thousands of compounds, and as new, more sensitive analytical tools evolve, it is quite certain that new constituents of urine will be recognized.' So it is a proven fact that our urine contains thousands of beneficial ingredients. Among the many urine constituents mentioned in Dr. Free's treatise is the following list of nutrients:

Nutritent	Amount per day
Alanine, total	38 mg
Arginine,	32 mg
Ascorbic acid	30 mg
Allantoin	12 mg

Amino acids, total	2.1 g
Bicarbonate	140 mg
Biotin	35 mg
Calcium	23 mg
Creatinine	1.4 mg
Cystine	120 mg
Dopamine	0.40 mg
Epinephrine	0.01 mg
Folic acid	4 mg
Glucose	100 mg
Glutamic acid	308 mg
Glycine	455 mg
Inositol	14 mg
Iodine	0.25 mg
Iron	0.5 mg
Lysine	56 mg
Magnesium	100 mg
Manganese	0.5 mg
Methionine	10 mg
Nitrogen	15 g
Ornithine	10 mg
Pantothenic acid	3 mg
Phenylalanine	21 mg
Phosphorus, organic	9 mg
Potassium	2.5 mg
Proteins	5 mg
Riboflavin	0.9 mg
Tryptophan	28 mg
Tyrosine	50 mg

Urea	24.5 mg
Vitamin B6	100 mg
Vitamin B12	0.03 mg
Zinc	1.4 mg

SOME IMPORTANT SUBSTANCES FOUND IN URINE

Substance	Qualities
Urokinase	Prevents the formation of blood clots in the blood vessels and is even capable of dissolving clots already formed.
Erythropoietine	Stimulates the bone marrow to increase the rate of production of erythrocytes (red blood corpuscles). Effective against anaemia.
Adrenaline and cortisol	Renders calming effect on stress.
Allantoin	Promotes wound healing.
Amino Acids	The building blocks from which proteins are made.
Ammonia	Prevents and eliminates skin conditions.
Anti toxin	Capable of neutralising the same toxin that stimulated the body to produce it.
Ascorbic acid (vitamin C)	Gives energy, prevents flu /colds and damage that leads to the weakening of the immune system.
Calcium	Essential for healthy bones and many vital functions. The most important and abundant element in the body.

Cortisone (natural)	Heals skin problems, calming effect on stress. Also useful against asthma and allergies. (Synthetic version has many side effects).
DHEA	Anti-cancer, anti-obesity and anti-aging properties.
Factor S	Induces sleep safely and naturally.
Hydrogen Peroxide	Has a powerful oxidising effect. Controls and kills bacteria, funguses, parasites and any other anaerobic organism it comes into contact with. Strengthens the immune system.
H-11	Inhibits the growth of cancer cells.
Magnesium	Effective against many diseases.
Melatonin	Balances moods. Strengthens the immune system, controls obesity and has anti-aging properties.
Phosphorus	Aids metabolism.
Renin	Maintains vascular tone. Useful against high blood pressure.
Urea	Facilitates the passage of bodily fluids, cellular waste, nutrients and oxygen through the skin. Balances blood pressure, skin moisturiser, improves glaucoma, combats tuberculosis.
Uric acid	Controls free radicals. Anti-aging properties.

Practical urine therapy

INTERNAL USE

Drinking fresh urine

Morning urine is the best. Take it from the mid-stream. You can start with a few drops, building up to one or more cups per day. Good as a tonic, as a preventative and to counter major and minor illnesses. If you don't want to swallow the urine, simply swill it around under the tongue for a few seconds and spit it out again, this will stimulate a powerful lymphatic response. Drinking a tablespoon of eight-day-old urine is a remarkably powerful way to beat bacterial and parasitic infections in the throat and often only takes one dose to completely cure the condition.

Sublingual

Take just one or two drops of urine under the tongue or in one of the ears every two hours or less. Using a dropper bottle is a good idea or if it is not available readily, urinate on to one of your fingers briefly and put it under the tongue. This method stimulates the part of the lymphatic system located under around the neck area and should not be underestimated as a highly effective healing technique

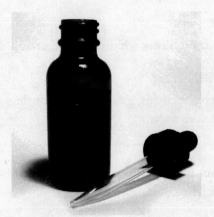

**Fig. 4.1 A dropper bottle can be used for
the sublingual method of urine therapy**

called 'The Universal Remedy' by Martin Lara in his book of the
same name (see the Bibliography section).

Fasting

Drink most of the urine you pass during the day. You can also take
some extra water. The urine will quickly change its taste into almost
neutral. Fasting on urine and water cleanses the blood. In this process
toxins are removed through the liver, skin and breath. This is a very
powerful technique and can lead to miraculous results in a very short
space of time.

Gargle

Gargling with urine works wonders when you have a sore throat. It
is also helps with toothache.

Enemas

Urine enemas and rectal implants work quickly in cleansing the colon
and in providing a direct immune system stimulant. Ideally use 4-8
days old urine mixed with some boiling hot water until it is warm
enough to be comfortably used in an enema.

Vaginal douche

Helpful with yeast problems, white discharge, etc.

Ear & eye drops

Ear infections; conjunctivitis, glaucoma etc. For the eyes, dilute the urine with some pure water.

Nasal wash

Particularly useful for sinusitis and other nasal problems (see the Exercise section: Yoga: Nasal cleansing).

Injection

A very powerful method of administering urine, especially used in emergency cases such as during serious infections and advanced cancer, although has been used to completely cure a wide range of diseases and health problems.

EXTERNAL USE

Massaging/Rubbing

You can use either fresh or old urine. Old urine (four to eight days) is generally more effective, but unfortunately, it has a strong smell. Massaging the whole body is a very important complementary treatment during fasting. It nourishes the body through the skin and helps against increased heartbeat. You can leave the urine on or wash it off after an hour or so with water or with a mild, natural soap. Massaging fresh (or more effectively stale) urine gives a beautifully soft skin. It is also very helpful and healing many kinds of skin problems, including itching, sunburns, eczema, psoriasis and acne.

Footbaths

Any skin and nail problems of the feet (athletes foot, ringworm etc.)

Mixing urine with hot water and soaking the feet for half and hour is also an excellent way of introducing urine into the system if you can't face drinking it directly as it is absorbed through the pores in the skin.

Compress

When rubbing is not appropriate, this is another way of applying urine on the skin. Wrap a flannel or rag in urine (preferably 4-8 days old) and wrap around the affected area (for instance over varicose veins or around a wounded elbow). Make sure to keep it moist.

Hair and scalp massage

Renders the hair soft, vibrant and clean. Sometimes stimulates new hair growth. Mix some urine (preferably 4-8 days old) with a small amount of hot water and pour over your head. Massage thoroughly into the scalp, dab excess urine off with some kitchen towel roll and leave on for at least half an hour for maximum effect.

Urine can also be used in place of regular shampoo. Simply pee into a suitable container before having a shower and pour the urine over the head whilst massaging it into the hair and scalp. Wash your hair with water after you've finished washing your body.

Some benefits of urine therapy

- ➤ A drastic boost to the immune system
- ➤ Painless purging of accumulated toxins
- ➤ Radiant, soft skin
- ➤ Shining eyes
- ➤ A balancing effect on the body (homeostasis)
- ➤ A general lift in mood
- ➤ Quantum healing of many diseases
- ➤ Improved memory
- ➤ Improved creativity
- ➤ Seemingly miraculous recovery from disease
- ➤ Improved meditation practice
- ➤ Free and regularly available

Urine facts

- One of the secrets of military survival training is that a soldier can live for a month or more without food or water, simply by drinking his own urine. A solider can also survive the effects of a biochemical attack by wrapping a urine soaked rag around his mouth.

- There are a number of advanced yogis living in the Himalayas who are reported to be well over 300 years of age. One method that some of them use to achieve such amazing health is by drinking and rubbing urine into their skin every day.

- The main ingredient of the amniotic fluid (the fluid that the foetus grows in) is urine.

- Fourcroy, the father of modern chemistry, wrote in 1801 "Human urine is not the product of evolution of man, on the contrary, the evolution of man is the product of his urine".

- Urine is a living, organic substance that is more powerful than antibiotics or chemotherapy for fighting and curing cancer.

> Urine has been the most investigated substance in the history of modern science. Research is done to find and isolate the specific urine ingredients that have disease-fighting properties. Once isolated, they are mass produced chemically, given an impressive name, encapsulated and sold at an unreasonably inflated price.

> Urine contains more than a dozen ingredients that fight cancer at all its stages of development. Some fight cancer tumours and others prevent the formation of free radicals. Most importantly, urine reactivates the lymphatic system to eliminate all cellular faeces from the lymphatic nodes, the birthplace of cancer.

> Natural foods and drinks produce clear urine that tastes fine the morning after.

> Urine therapy is probably simplest, cheapest, most powerful and most universal healing system.

> Everyone can benefit from urine regardless of age, sex, race, status, geographical location and affliction.

> The former prime minister of India, Morarji Desai was an enthusiastic proponent of urine therapy. In 1978, during an interview on 60 minutes, he said 'In America your scientists are preparing extracts from urine for heart trouble…your people are drinking other people's urine but not their own. And it costs dollars, thousands of dollars, while theirs is free and more effective.'

> In February 1996, hundreds of scientists and doctors began a global conference devoted to what organisers say is a potential cure for a host of killer diseases including AIDS – human urine. Nearly 600 delegates from 17 nations gathered in the capital of the western Indian state of Goa for the first World Conference on Auto-Urine Therapy.

A personal account
from Sari

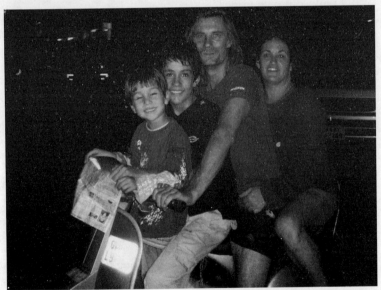

Fig. 4.2 Sari with her family on their scooter in Goa.

'In Shivambu Kapla Vidhi, which is part of the Damar Tantra, Lord
Shiva is explaining to his wife Parvati the procedure and rules to
drinking one's own urine to overcome illness and a weak mind.

I never came across those scriptures but was lucky enough to sit by a group of people in Patnem beach, Goa and hear a conversation about colloidal silver and the Watercure. I was given an issue of 'Insider Goa' magazine and quickly educated myself on the benefits of using colloidal silver, of drinking enough water daily and of using sea or rock salt instead of the common poisonous white table salt. These were all enlightening facts with success stories of users, yet I felt that there must be something inside all of us, that we must posses the power and knowledge to help ourselves – by ourselves.

'Drink your pee,' this guy said.

'What?' I shifted my whole attention towards him.

'Drink your own urine!!!'

I felt that the exclamation marks at the end of the last sentence would go on and on forever.

'Explain!' I demanded. And so he did.

The next morning I was there in the bathroom collecting my piss in a cup. I held it with my hands, feeling the warmth in my palms and smelling odours I chose not to judge.

It is now six months since that first cup went down my throat and through my body and I felt as lucky as Parvati to discover such a wonderful secret, such an amazing therapy, such a taste. The first changes were quite subtle. The first changes took place deep inside me. I felt positive. I felt happy. I felt quiet.

I was getting up at 5am and after drinking my own urine I was sitting down quietly meditating. I wasn't feeling guilty that I was only doing five or ten minutes of meditation. On the contrary I felt like praising myself for doing the minimum, which for me was the maximum of the moment.

Sitting for meditation gradually grew longer each day and so was my strength. The discipline to improve my diet, to look after myself became stronger. I joined yoga classes, which I adore, and I observe what my body is doing, where my soul is heading and it makes me feel like I am in ecstasy sometimes. I touch my conditioner and shampoo free hair and I apply the external application of urine for improving my hair, my skin, and my teeth.

I can go on and on talking about urine therapy but I stop now and urge you, who found my account exciting, to read more about urine therapy, to study it, to do it and see for yourselves. There are many websites with much information about it.

The line of thought I always support is to stop judging before knowing.

> Hear.
> Try.
> Experiment.
> Conclude.
> Drink and be merry!

- Sari Horton, November 2005

MY COMMENTS ON SARI'S ACCOUNT

Sari is a mother of two boys, Ram and Orin and is married to Chris, a guitar-maker and teacher. The family live in Goa, India. I met Sari in May 2005 and she seemed quite sceptical about urine therapy but interested never the less. I like to tell people about urine therapy and natural healthcare and Sari was obviously keen to learn about such things.

The 'Insider Goa' magazine, she mentioned was a publication I was editing at the time, which regularly featured articles about issues connected with the Five Point Plan as well as Indian culture. I believe that the simple combination of:

> ➢ Correcting hydration and salt levels in the body
> ➢ Correcting core dietary and lifestyle habits
> ➢ Utilising one's own urine therapeutically

It is so important to humanity in general, that it is well worth promoting (even if the advice, publications and pamphlets that I produce don't make any profit). The magazine lost money and was discontinued after just over a year, however many people commented on how the simple advice they had read had drastically improved their health; especially the articles on WaterCure, Colloidal Silver and Urine Therapy.

Sari was enthusiastic about homeopathy when I first met her, however if the body is unintentionally and chronically dehydrated, the benefits of homeopathic preparations will be short-lived at best. The same is true of other holistic healing modalities, such as acupressure, acupuncture, chiropractic, herbalism, reiki, yoga therapy, magnet therapy, reflexology, vitamin and mineral supplements etc.

An on-going theme in my conversations with other holistic practitioners is this simple point, nicely put by Dr.Batmanghelidj:

'Water is the cash-flow of the body. Don't bankrupt yourself'

Q&A

Isn't urine a toxic body waste?

Urine is a blood by-product and though it contains small amounts of body waste, never so much as to cause any damage.

Wouldn't it be harmful to put those toxins back into the body?

The toxins found within urine are not enough to be toxic to the body from which it came. Anything that was in your blood cannot be harmful to the person where it came from. Had it been that harmful, that person would already be dead. Besides, the urine you drink does not go directly to the blood stream; first it goes into the digestive system where its ingredients are sorted out.

What about people claiming that drinking urine will cause cirrhosis of the liver and harm or paralyse the kidneys?

They have a misconception with respect to drinking urine and what role the intestines play in urine therapy. The liver removes toxic waste and dumps it at the beginning of the small intestine to aid in the process of digestion. The urine a person drinks goes into the same spot where the liver discharges this cellular waste, but the toxins urine contains are a very small amount in comparison to what the liver dumps at the same site. Always drink the correct amount of pure water each day.

Is there a way to purify the body to improve the taste of urine before starting to drink it?

At first, some people experience nausea, headaches and other strong reactions before they get used to it and start seeing any results. Do not despair or give up. Remember that urine is a sample of what is flowing through your veins and repulsive urine should be a motivation to improve the internal conditions, rather than an excuse for not continuing with urine therapy. Cut down on heavily salted, meaty or artificial foods and drink a bare minimum of two litres of pure water each day. Three to four litres per day is ideal for most physically active medium to heavy weight people. If you are drinking some of your first pee of the day, you will find it much more pleasant tasting if you have remembered to have a decent drink of water before sleeping.

Can a girl drink her urine during the menstrual cycle?

Yes, a girl can drink her urine during menstruation. The urethra and the vagina are two different organs. It is also worth noting that there is nothing in the menstruation fluid that can cause harm if you accidentally drink a little of it mixed with the urine.

Can a person drink his urine while on medications?

There is the possibility of overdosing on a particular medication by recycling the portion of it discharged in the urine. Hormone supplements can be taken while drinking your urine however you should frequently monitor your hormone intake because as the affected organ improves, the supplement you need has to be reduced accordingly. Generally speaking, it is fine to drink your urine whilst on medications but if you are unsure, start with the sublingual method, which is safe in all circumstances.

Does the medical profession recognize urine therapy?

Yes and no. Yes, urine is mentioned more than any other substance in the Hippocratic texts and there are countless scientific studies proving its effectiveness. No, you will be unlikely to hear about it from your doctor or through the mainstream press.

Is any urine fine or must it be my own?

Your own urine is perfect, your particular health needs, however in very serious cases where the patient is unable to urinate, the urine of a relative or friend can be used (perhaps sublingually or as a sub-coetaneous injection). Baby's urine is generally the purest.

Can urine be mixed with other drinks to hide the flavour?

Yes, some people mix their urine with fruit juice or water; however it is better to drink your urine pure if you possibly can. There is no better way of educating yourself about the state of your body than by drinking your own fresh, undiluted urine and remember that when the correct foods and plenty of water are taken it should not taste bad at all.

What sort of doses do people take?

It varies from a couple of drops under the tongue (sublingually), after every two hours to litres per day, depending on what your aims are. A yogi who is living off a small bowl of rice each day may well be drinking the majority of all the urine he passes, possibly adding up to many litres per day. Regularity of intake is more important than quantity.

Won't it make my breath smell?

Quite possibly, especially if you are not drinking enough water through the day. I recommend giving your teeth a brush with non-fluoridated toothpaste after drinking urine.

Urine therapy & Natural Hygiene

The Natural Hygiene movement (called the Nature Cure movement in Europe) developed around the early 1800's and was a sizable revolt against the medical practices of the time. Pioneers such as Dr. Herbert Shelton exposed the drug-medical approach as nothing less than a completely false doctrine from start to finish. I have been greatly influenced by the many public domain books that are now available free of charge online and its philosophy of not trying to 'cure' illness symptoms but rather removing the cause of it and allowing the body to overcome the problem naturally.

I asked some Natural Hygiene practitioners and enthusiasts about their opinions concerning urine therapy and got the following responses:

'This is my current opinion': Everything we eat contains nutrients, toxins and inert stuff (fibres). We always want to choose whatever contains lots of nutrients, and fibre and avoid the toxins. E.g. a chocolate bar may have a lot of nutrients, but probably more toxins. A carrot may have lots of nutrients & fibre, and minimal toxins (but note that sugar & starches can behave as toxins in some people). Urine may have some nutrients, but probably more toxins.

Since it is toxic garbage coming out of the body. Toxin level probably varies from day to day.

So, what do we do with those foods that contain both nutrients and toxins? I think, if the toxins go over a certain limit say 2% we better avoid them. Why? Because the body MUST remove the toxins first, it is an emergency! So all (vital) energy goes to toxin-removal, and the nutrients are ignored. Possibly, some nutrients may get attention, after the fire brigade has put out all the fires.

How does it feel like, when the fire-brigade speeds out the gate? We feel stimulated! Like we have lots of energy. But instead we are depleting our battery too fast, and this will probably come back and hit us later, when we get very tired and sleepy, and may need new stimulants to stay awake.

'So, I can imagine, drinking urine may make us feel stimulated, perhaps even dizzy, we may feel stronger and more energetic - but it is all an illusion, the 'stimulant delusion'.

- Anna

'No offence, and just my humble opinion, but anyone who would drink urine is an I-D-I-O-T.'

- Gary S

'It is important to consult our instincts on such notions as drinking one's urine, (assuming that they are intact). Instinctively... the vast majority of people know that the idea of drinking waste products that the body has gone through considerable effort to eliminate through its normal channels, is, as Gary says, 'idiotic' i.e. something that someone with their senses intact would not employ. Beyond that, instinctively the vast majority of us just feel plain old revulsion at the notion.

Do we need to convince a sane person to drink pure water, to breathe pure air or to seek out sunlight? No, again, these things are instinctive. For those, whose educated mind has gotten in the way we can present to them scientific data supporting breathing, drinking water and acquiring sunlight but it is a sad reflection on us that we often need to do so.'

- Dr. Paul Goldberg, MPH, DC, DACBN

'In support of Dr Golberg, Gary and Anna, I consider the utilisation of any waste product of our bodies as going against all human instinct. All animals in their natural state not only do not do so, they will not eat any food which has been contaminated by urine or faecal matter.'

- John L. Fielder, D.O, N.D:

'According to my understanding the Hygienist would rely only upon those substances that have a normal healthy relation to the body, fresh air, sunshine, fresh water etc. Urea being a waste product cannot be classified as food, therefore the only healthy relationship it has with the body is when it is passed. Reintroducing a non-food, already passed, cannot serve any useful purpose. In fact it is the 'Wisdom' of the body, in its never-ending trek to a higher state of health, that removed the substance in the first place.

Therefore, we would have to conclude that Urine drinking is not normal healthy activity, and should not be part of the Hygienic Lifestyle.'

- Karl Anderson

'At last we are getting some intelligent responses I was beginning to despair. Anybody who even contemplates putting back into the body that which it has excreted for a valid reason, does not understand 'toxemia, the basic cause of disease'. Without that understanding, the Hygienic teachers will never get through to you.'

- Peter

The Natural Hygienist's objections to urine therapy were unanimous yet I was unconvinced by their responses. My reply was:

'Thanks Anna for your balanced response. Yes, toxins are present in urine (called 'Shivambu' or 'water of Shiva' in India) however this doesn't necessarily make it a waste product. Rather than being 'toxic', urine (which is about 95% water) may actually contain some of the purest water that we can drink. It is a by-product of our blood, filtered by the liver and kidneys. The cleaner the blood is, the healthier the urine will be. Urine is pure, fresh, organic, live, filtered 'structured' water, at body temperature, containing large quantities of pure, pre-digested nutrients. Urine therapists would answer that urine ingestion promotes a state of homeostasis amongst other benefits. The practice goes back thousands of years and is detailed in the Damar Tantra, where lord Shiva extols the benefits – both spiritual and physical - to his divine consort Parvati.'

Excerpts:

'Shivambu (auto- urine) is heavenly nectar, which is capable of destroying senility and diseases… He who has continued the practice for twelve years will live so long as the moon and the stars last. He is not troubled by dangerous animals such as snakes, and no poisons can kill him. He cannot be consumed by fire, and can float on water just like wood… The Yogi who follows these instructions achieves pre-eminence among all Yogis, and his movements become totally unrestricted. He acquires the strength of a thousand elephants, and is able to obtain (and digest) any food which he desires.'

I like the fire-engine example however it doesn't convince me in the case of urine. It's more than just feeling stronger and more energetic. The benefits are spiritually, mentally and emotionally tangible as well. In a nutshell, my understanding of the ancient practice is that we are all God (if only we knew it) and the urine that flows from us contains divine properties that can help lead to 'attaining divinity whilst in the physical body'.

If that makes me an I.D.I.O.T (thanks Gary) then so be it.

'Instinctively', we don't do many things that would benefit others and ourselves, such as applying the necessary discipline to undergo intense spiritual practices like meditation and chanting mantras for example. Believe it or not, there are people in India, especially in the Himalayas, who are physically immortal and never need to eat or drink anything. They can indeed fly around the place, vanish in a ball of light and reappear on the other side of the world, heal people with a glance etc and have been doing so for a very long time.

Does hygiene take 'revelation' into account? There may be more to this practice of urine therapy than you give credit for, however I reserve the right to be wrong. It's true I'm interested in, which is why I am so enamoured with Natural Hygiene. The Natural Hygiene movement is, I believe a developing art and shunning anything that does not fit neatly with the basic principles may not be the best way forward.

John, you say that all animals do not drink their urine instinctively however I've watched video footage of a monkey peeing into his mouth and he seems very happy. And what about toddlers who instinctively want to drink out of their potty?

Dr. Goldberg, it's no doubt true to say that 'the vast majority of us just feel plain old revulsion at the notion of drinking urine'. It's also true to say that most of us are chronically dehydrated, which means the urine is faecal-extracted and tastes terrible. It's also true to say that just because most people don't want to do something, doesn't mean that certain something is against God's laws.

Urine therapy & cancer

Dr. Joseph Eldor, MD wrote an interesting paper called 'Urotherapy for patients with cancer' and I've included a simplified overview of it below. The full paper can be found at: www.csen.com/theory/cancer.htm

ABSTRACT

Cancer cells release various antigens.

Some of these antigens are contained in the patient's urine.

Urine therapy provides the intestinal lymphatic system with these antigens, against which antibodies may be produced.

These antibodies may be transpierced through the blood stream and attack the tumour at the cellular level.

PHILOSOPHY OF CANCER

Microbes were known long before the germ theory of disease emerged.

It was not the germ theory that revolutionised medicine but

rather it was the philosophy of the germ theory that revolutionised medicine by making germs the scapegoat for disease.

Most human cancers lack truly tumour specific antigens.

The same neoplastic cell can express several different tumour antigens.

At this point, the author gives a very scientific analysis of tumour antigens in urine.

PRECONCLUSION

Slegeris said 'The problem of cancer…is not merely a biological and laboratory problem, but belongs to a certain to the realm of philosophy…All experiments require certain philosophical preparation. And I have the feeling that in the case of cancer, many experiments were undertaken without the necessary philosophical background and therefore proved useless".

CONCLUSION

Urine therapy is a valid for of immunotherapy for cancer patients.

It is better than clonal immunotherapy because the patient's urine contains the many tumour antigens that comprise the tumour.

Drinking urine provides the intestinal lymphatic system with the tumour antigens against which they produce antibodies due to non-self recognition.

Antibodies are transpierced through the blood stream and the tumour at its cells.

Testimonies

'In one of my own experiments, I prepared the Ultimate Universal Remedy (sublingual urine) for a child who was suffering with epilepsy, asthma, mental retardation and clumsiness for more than 10 years, having at least one epileptic fit every day. I instructed the family to apply the 4 drops of diluted urine under the tongue every 2 to 3 hours while the child was awake. I also advised them to open the window a little while he slept and that he be given trace minerals. He started improving immediately and after the third day he had no more epileptic seizures. I checked back with the family in South America and a few months later the child was doing great'.

- Martin Lara,

'I started drinking a cup of urine every morning about a month ago and I have to say it has done wonders for me, not least higher energy levels and a much better complexion'.

- Daniel, London

'Whilst on holiday in Hawaii earlier this year, I cut my knee on some rocks when I was swimming in some rough waters. It was a really bad injury and I soon had septicemia, staphococys and blood poisoning. My leg looked terrible with blood and pus pouring out of it. I tried everything I could think of to alleviate the condition, including Eccinasia, Grapefruit, colloidal silver, swabs and drinking my own urine but nothing seemed to work, even though they gave temporary relief. The local people told me I was in serious trouble, which made me even more determined to find a solution. Eventually, I tried an injection of 1cc of fresh urine into the sub-cutaneous tissue around my front quadriceps. Within 12 hours of the first injection, my condition was 50% better. After the second injection on the second day it was 75% better and after 8 injections everything is completely fine again, all I have left is a small bruise where the needle went (I had to use a vets needle the first time!). As a great bonus, an old pain in my right ear, which a doctor told me 20 years ago was a cancer, has disappeared'.

- Tony, London

'Urine makes me feel wonderful. The more I drink, the better I feel and the less inclined I am to eat junk food. I feel much more creative, I have more energy and I've even noticed that my singing voice has got better!'

- Jane, London

'Thanks for your advice about the urine therapy. Is it a coincidence that since starting of 'the' cure I have not had to use any cream on my itchy legs even though they had been bitten to pieces two days ago by 'who knows what' whilst spreading manure? 'Why on earth is she soaking her feet in urine!?' my friends asked. Well, they feel better already. Lots of positive signs seem to be going on. We really are amazed!'

- Jemma, Norwich

'Pedro Alvarez' body was invaded by amoebas 10 years earlier and he was suffering the corresponding discomforts since then. Alvarez collected his urine one night and kept it in the bathroom for about 15 hours, then drank it the next day. By misunderstanding the instructions of a friend, who told him to drink fresh urine, he accidentally discovered a new application of urine therapy for amoebas and tapeworms. Surprisingly, 15-hour-old urine did not taste that bad, he explains, but he immediately drank a tall glass of juice because he felt strange. Within 10 minutes or so he had abundant diarrhoea. Alvarez was forced to stay close to the bathroom for the next two days. The diarrhoea was so bad that he feared dehydration, but he knew to drink a lot of water with a pinch of sea salt. He spent the weekend at home drinking water and diluted fresh fruit juice. Monday morning he went back to work almost completely recovered. Three years later he hadn't had any more amoeba-related problems. Apparently the fermented urine of a person with parasites is so effective that it even removes the eggs of these parasites.'

- From Martin Lara's book 'Uropathy'.

Summary

Urine has been used across the world for thousands of years as a powerful healing elixir. Far from being a waste product, urine can be used as an entire system for diagnosis and treatment for even the most serious diseases. Urine is very possibly the most powerful holistic remedy. Most people are not aware of this fact because the very nature of urine therapy is that it is free and uncontrollable, therefore there is little incentive for its promotion in the media and through doctors in surgeries.

DIET

Introduction

Until the age of about eighteen I was a willing victim of modern day food advertising. Preferring to eat microwave burger and chips, cheese and ham sandwiches and baked beans on toast, I shunned my mother's cooking and would often avoid family meals in favour of quickly zapping a '90-second beef burger' from the freezer or making a sandwich comprising of bleached white bread, horrifically de-natured margarine, processed cream cheese and a couple of slices of processed ham. I now smile when I look back at my appalling diet, born of laziness, ignorance and social conditioning. I thought that I loved my harmful snacks; indeed I virtually lived off them completely, yet I now know that those 'delicious' snacks did not love me! Indeed it was a highly abusive relationship.

I sometimes wondered why I had pimples on my forehead and around my nose, or why every few weeks I'd have a 'terrible time' on the toilet, experiencing brief yet fiercely intense periods of pain as I struggled with constipation. I'd ask my parents why I sometimes got constipated but they couldn't answer my question correctly because they hadn't learned about nutrition. They simply replied that 'lots of people get constipated sometimes'. When I asked about the spots, my father would joke that it was 'God's way of bringing teenagers down a peg or two'! Of course the real answers were simple; that I was living off dangerous junk food and not drinking nearly enough pure water. It wasn't until I spent two months travelling in India with a close friend (who was very knowledgeable about nutrition) that I learned some practical truths about my diet.

I learned that I didn't need to eat meat to be happy. India is a largely vegetarian country and I was told to avoid eating any meat as it would probably give me some kind of food poisoning, so I didn't take any meat for two months and felt much better for it. I felt so much better in fact that I soon became a vegetarian. My travelling companion suggested that I should spend three months adhering to the 'Hay System' of health, which advocates not mixing proteins and carbohydrates in the same meal and eating whole foods. He said that after three months I might experience a slight 'healing response' (headaches, mood swings, nausea etc) but that was because the core, deep tissue toxins would be being expelled at that time and that actually was a good thing. I'll never forget that 'slight' healing response; it was horrific! Luckily it only lasted for three days but after those three days of 'purgatory', I vowed never to fill my body with low quality food again. It was an easy decision, as I never would wish such an experience even on my worst enemy. An excerpt from my diary at the time read:

'I feel like a million evil substances are pouring out of my skin! Whatever it is that is coming out is foul…it hurts! Whatever it is – is disgusting! I itch all over and it's very painful, all I can do is stay in the house and lie down or watch TV – can't face going out. If I laugh, cough or simply tense my muscles the itching becomes unbearable. I had a hot bath this afternoon but got out a few minutes later because my whole body erupted into intense itching, I couldn't stand it, must be the heat making the toxins come out quicker. I'm waking up every few hours during the night and scratching myself –sometimes under the arms, sometimes the legs, sometime my groin…I hope this ends soon because I'm not sure I can stand it anymore!'

Those three days did indeed occur after about three months after stating my new dietary regime. Following the diet that my friend had prescribed I was eating a large fruit salad every morning, drinking lots of water, not mixing a protein with a carbohydrate in the same meal and eating lots of organic brown rice (sometimes simply as a meal on it's own with a bit of organic tamari sauce), mung bean soups and salads. It is interesting to note that in the yogic tradition, mung beans have been referred to by yogis as 'food of the gods', I guess because of their purifying nature. Apart from my three days of healing response, I felt marvellous. My skin became clear and shiny, my eyes were bright and every morning I would wake up completely clear headed and energised. Everyone said how quickly I had changed from a slightly over-weight, slightly spotty person to a figure of health and vitality and I was so happy to have applied the discipline to change my diet; it was one of the best decisions I've ever made. The only problem with this Hay system was that I started losing a lot of weight and became skinny; I felt like a million dollars but didn't want to continue losing weight.

That was about fourteen years ago and my knowledge has increased since then. Now I know how to obtain optimum nutrition, optimum health and vitality without ending up too skinny or without having to go through such a disturbing healing response. This chapter provides some essential information needed to achieve excellent results in the fields of personal health and healing.

'Let your food be your medicine and your medicine be your food.'

- Hippocrates

A closer look at diet

Degraded, chemicalised, pre-packaged food is damaging to the health for many reasons, yet the vast majority of food available in the West fits into this category. When we walk down a supermarket aisle we are confronted with myriad choices of brightly coloured packages and cartons, but how many of us actually take the time to study the ingredients on the back and make an informed decision about whether or not it is healthy or unhealthy?

The reading list and Internet sites at the back of this book give details of some excellent books and online resources concerning the various aspects of healthy eating. Factors of key importance to consider regarding diet are:

> Is this food natural, or has it been degraded in some way?

> What are the nutritional benefits of this food and how easy is it to digest?

> What is the quantity of foods being eaten?

In this chapter the reader will learn how to live far more healthily by eating a smaller amount of primarily whole food and practicing fasting once in a while. Back in the days when I was eating junk and fast food it seemed like an impossible task to change my diet and live in a truly healthy way, yet in hindsight I now realise I was totally wrong in my attitude. I have learned that the healthiest diet is the simplest, cheapest and most pleasant. The diet outlined in this chapter does not require spending hours in the kitchen preparing complicated recipes, washing up copious pots and pans, forking out lots of money on expensive ingredients or eating bland, flavourless food. On the contrary, this diet is so easy to prepare that a child can follow it.

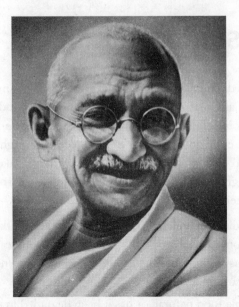

Fig. 5.1 Mahatma Gandhi

'Though I have had two serious illnesses in my life, I believe that man has little need to drug himself. 999 cases out of a thousand can be brought round by means of a well-regulated diet, water & earth treatment and similar household remedies.'

- Mahatma Ghandi

Whole food

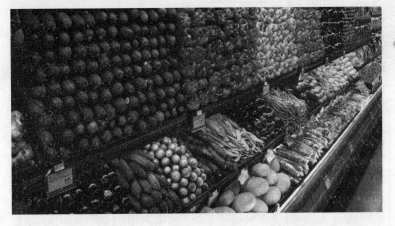

Fig. 5.2 Healthy, wholesome, raw food - just as nature intended

Whole food can be defined as:

'Naturally occurring food that has not been tampered with'.

In fitting with the holistic view of life and health, it is important to incorporate whole food into the diet. The following chart gives a simple overview of which foods to avoid and which to increase:

Increase	Decrease
Raw foods	Cooked foods
Organic foods	Non-organic foods
Salad (fruit and vegetable)	Pre-packaged, commercial food
Juices	Cooked grains, bread, pasta
Soaked and sprouted nuts/seeds	Caffeine, alcohol, sugary drinks
Superfoods	Animal products

COMPONENTS OF WHOLE FOOD

The human body utilises food for two main reasons:

> As fuel for energy

> As raw material to help repair itself

It is via the processes of digestion, food is broken down and transported throughout the blood stream into the cells of the body.

The following table overviews the various components of whole food and how they benefit us:

COMPONENT	DESCRIPTION	SOURCE EXAMPLES
Fibre	The indigestible part of plant matter. Facilitates the passage of food through the digestive system and absorbs harmful substances.	Oats, carrots, wholemeal bread, rice, banana, pinto beans

Proteins	Nitrogen containing compounds. Necessary for building muscle tissue and repairing cells. The breakdown of proteins into amino acids leaves nitrogenous waste, which must later be eliminated by the body.	Dairy products, fish, meat, kidney beans, sunflower seeds, spirulina, nuts
Fats	Provide the body with energy and enables it to store vital fat-soluble vitamins such as A, D, E & K. The body also needs fats to cushion the internal organs and create myelin sheaths (insulation) around the nerves.	Dairy products, fish, meat, oils, soya beans, olives, nuts, avocado
Carbohydrates	The main energy source for the human body. Simple carbohydrates can be completely broken down whereas more complex cannot be digested and these act like fibre, helping to kept the digestive system healthy.	Wholemeal bread, potatoes, rice, pasta, chick peas
Vitamins and Minerals	Essential for the correct functioning of all bodily processes. Plants take in minerals from the soil and vitamins. Exposing food to heat (cooking) destroys many vitamins and minerals.	Fruit, vegetables

Life force from the sun makes its way into our bodies via plants (photosynthesis), which are then eaten by us. Eating meat and dairy is merely a 'second hand' way of receiving this energy.

THE VALUE OF WHOLE FOODS

Having a basic knowledge, the nutritional value of the different foods can help when deciding what exactly you are going to eat. 'Healing with Whole Foods' by Paul Pitchford is an excellent treatise on the healing properties of whole foods and has a comprehensive index system, making a thorough knowledge of each food easy to learn (see Bibliography section).

The following chart gives a brief overview of the health benefits of some of the most popular whole foods.

Apple	Reduces risk of heart attack and stroke and helps bowel movement thanks to its fibre content. Flavanoids act as anti-oxidants, which combat free radicals.
Banana	Helps to prevent high blood pressure and protect against atherosclerosis thanks to its potassium content. Help to activate the cells that compose the stomach lining, so they produce a thicker protective mucus barrier against stomach acids.
Blackcurrant	Only 6 blackcurrants contain the same amount of vitamin C as a large lemon.

Almond nut	Antioxidant benefits of the vitamin E contained in Almonds. Also contains healthy fats, magnesium and potassium aiding all round health.
Sunflower seed	Contains high levels of vitamins E and B1, manganese, magnesium, copper and other nutrients. Sunflower seeds also have a very high oil content and are an excellent source of polyunsaturated oil.
Broccoli	Rich with Calcium, vitamin C, vitamin A, antioxidants and fibre contributing to all round health and cancer prevention.
Carrot	The beta carotene in carrots turns to large doses of vitamin A which helps to protect against cardiovascular disease and cancer as well as promoting good vision, especially night vision.
Spinach	Its high levels of vitamins A, B2, C and K along with manganese, magnesium, iron and potassium boost the health and can help to reverse illnesses such as osteoporosis, heart disease and cancer.

SOME BENEFITS OF A WHOLE FOOD DIET

➢ Enjoy better tasting food.

➢ Feel vibrant after eating rather than tired and groggy.

➢ Save money by avoiding unnecessary packaged foods.

➢ Become healthier with each meal.

➢ Give your body the correct nutrients it needs to function properly.

➢ Be protected against disease in the future.

➢ Enjoy a lighter, more joyous state of being.

> ➤ Fall asleep and wake up more easily.

> ➤ Not damaging to the environment.

FOOD FACTS

> ➤ Non-organic produce is grown in soil that has long since been spoiled with chemicals - rendering it nutritionally compromised.

> ➤ Eating healthily is cheaper than living off junk food.

> ➤ Meat products and meat-derived products are the leading cause of food poisoning cases around the world.

> ➤ A power-packed snack can be created by blending fruits or vegetables and drinking as a juice.

> ➤ Good health is more connected with the body's ability to assimilate the nutrients in the food than it is with the amount of nutritious food that is eaten. Less is often more.

> ➤ A 330ml can of Coke contains fifty grams of refined sugar (nine teaspoons).

> ➤ By eating an average of one packet of crisps each day, a total of five litres of refined vegetable oil is consumed during one year.

> ➤ Each year the average adult in Britain eats 15 pounds in weight of harmful food additives.

> ➤ Honey is the only food that humans eat that never goes rancid.

> ➤ Mayonnaise is capable of killing lice and acts as a hair conditioner.

> ➤ Coconut water can be used as a substitute for blood plasma. It is 'liquid endosperm' which means it surrounds the embryo and provides nutrition.

Q & A

Do I have to stop eating all junk food to get healthier?

No, although if you are sick it is a good idea completely clean up your eating habits, at least until you get better. Cutting out the really damaging foods and drinks and replacing them with healthy alternatives is a good start.

My child only likes junk food, what can I do?

Firstly, you can try to explain why living off junk food is a bad idea in a way that they can relate to. If they are teenaged, perhaps you can talk about how low quality food can cause spotty skin or if they are younger, perhaps let them see how much you enjoy eating healthy food and offer encouragement for them to follow your lead. Point out how many older people live with pain and disease because they have eaten bad food all their life and always promote the healthy=happy attitude. Of course, always try to prepare and provide quality, varied and tasty snacks/meals for your children. It doesn't have to be gourmet but it does have to taste better than the junk alternatives. Find out which junk foods in particular your child likes and look around for the best natural alternatives.

I really like junk food and don't think I'd enjoy healthy eating.

I suggest that you need to re-evaluate your attitudes and think more clearly about what 'enjoying' life is really about. It may take some effort at first to change bad eating habits but the results are always worth of it. You'll soon learn that healthy food can actually taste much better than junk food but you'll need to get your priorities in order first.

I live on a very low income, how can I afford to eat healthy food?

It can actually be cheaper to eat only healthy food. Being careful about what you buy, where you buy it from and when you buy it will always save you money. For instance, avoiding pre-packaged food and buying organic fruit and vegetables from a local box delivery scheme will save money as will eating seasonal, local produce and visiting the local supermarket half an hour before closing, to take advantage of the discounts on fresh foods that are approaching their sell-by date (but still within their use-by date).

There is so much contradictory advice about diet, how can I be sure what to believe?

Follow your instincts and take time to consider your diet carefully. Be aware that information coming from the mainstream media is often geared towards making profit and not necessarily correct. When looking at information presented to you, consider the following: Is someone selling something? Is someone trying to scare me? Does this information sound like the truth? Is it based on unbiased, real life people or is it the result of faceless research institutes and so-called experts?

Why is it important to eat slowly and chew your food well?

Chewing food thoroughly eases the burden on the digestive system, primarily by covering the food with saliva (which contains hydrogen peroxide).

In a nutshell, what guidelines can I follow to have a more healthy diet?

Avoid artificial and eat more natural foods. Always eat organic whenever possible and avoid all GM food. Less is more; skipping meals is healthy. The more you cook a food, the more you destroy its nutrients, so eating more raw food and less cooked food is a key part of the Five Point Plan.

SAMPLE HEALTHY SHOPPING LIST

- ➢ Oats
- ➢ Carrots, broccoli, garlic
- ➢ Apples, bananas, lemons
- ➢ Natural yoghurt
- ➢ Tahini
- ➢ Wholemeal crackers
- ➢ Extra virgin olive oil
- ➢ Sea salt
- ➢ Cayenne pepper
- ➢ Hemp seeds
- ➢ Mung beans (for sprouting or making into soup)
- ➢ Chick peas
- ➢ Mixed nuts

Vegetarian diet

In my opinion, people who claim to enjoy eating meat are deluding themselves and unknowingly subverting their mental, emotional and spiritual potential as human beings. Harsh words perhaps, but not as harsh as being slaughtered in a factory farm simply to end up on a plate as someone's dinner.

My old landlord had been a butcher all his life, from the age of thirteen until he retired (having built up a chain of butcher shops) aged seventy. By the age of eighty he was incontinent, crippled and cursed with the most explosive temper I've ever witnessed. He was a man who was consumed with hate for the world and although he lived only two hundred yards from the beautiful Dorset coast, he would brag that in the last fifteen years he not bothered to see the sea once. Another one of his quirks was to raise his zimmer frame as if to attack anyone who dared contradict him whilst shouting 'Shit Off!' and other words to that effect at the top of his voice.

During one of our conversations I asked him how much meat he had eaten in his life and he proudly proclaimed that he had not been a day without eating meat, apart from times that he had been ill in hospital. I asked him how he would feel if he was told that he had to stop eating it and he replied 'If I could never eat any meat again I would kill myself tomorrow'. Such is the effect that consuming flesh and blood can have upon us.

'What's meat got? It's got the lot!' exclaimed the UK TV adverts of the 1980's and the fallacy is still being promoted today in school classrooms and via marketing campaigns. The lie gets passed down through the generations, from parents and teachers to the impressionable children and only a small percentage of people ever take the time to consider the true implications of such an abominable habit.

The following poem is about how all our actions in daily life have a specific karmic effect; or more simply 'what goes around comes around'. The Hindu and Buddhist belief is that wars are the consequence of violent seeds sown by us all, such as killing animals unnecessarily for food.

SEEDS OF WAR

By Dasanu Dasa

We justify our selfish deeds,
Disguise our crimes as urgent needs,
Or pay another for their stealth,
In acts we won't perform ourselves.
"I'm innocent!" I hear you say.
The proof? Complicity every day,
In heinous deeds and murderous crime,
The violence starts at breakfast time.
Now, knife to throat I've never put,

And gentle man I am to boot!
We've often heard this alibi,
Then watched annihilation of a fly,
Who's only crime is was to pass,
Within range of our poison gas.

So comes the purpose of this rhyme,
To point out that this is a crime.
And though sanctioned by the laws of man,
God forbids this evil plan.
If innocence be there, indeed,
It's in the ones on whom we feed.
We send them to their awful fate,
Unseen until upon your plate.
Though horses, budgies, dogs and cats,
Were not put on earth for that.
So brothers, sisters, please be kind,
And do not kill these friends of mine.
For brothers and sisters all we be,
In God's great cosmic family.

But if these words you cannot hear,
And to my plea you will not yield,
My friends I see you're destined for,
The slaughterhouse of the battlefield.

Seeing as the vast majority of saints, sages and great teachers were/are staunch vegetarians, it never ceases to amaze me how many people feel justified in eating meat.

'Since all sentient beings are equal as my only son, how can I allow my followers to eat the flesh of my son? Eating meat to me is out of the question. I have never allowed, I am not allowing, and I will never allow this practice - I have strictly condemned eating meat in every way.'

- Buddha

'There is no beast on earth nor bird which flieth....but the same is a people like unto you. All God's creatures are God's family.'

- Qaran

'One is dearest to God who has no enemies among the living beings, who is non-violent to all creatures.'

- Krishna, Bhagavad Gita:

'For as long as men massacre animals, they will kill each other. Indeed, he who sows the seed of murder and pain cannot reap joy and love.'

- Pythagoras

'Primum non nocere.'

(First, do no harm)

- Hippocrates

'This is a lasting ordinance for the generations to come, wherever you live: You must not eat any fat or blood.'

- Leviticus 3:17 (Bible)

SOME REASONS WHY I FEEL WE SHOULD AVOID EATING MEAT

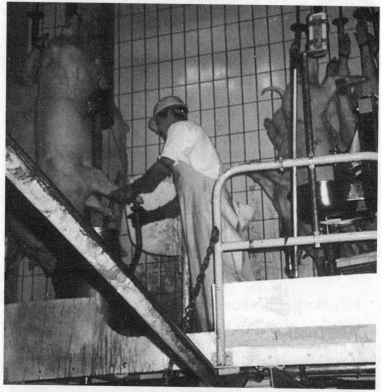

Fig. 5.3 A factory farmer busy processing mass slaughtered pigs

➤ Human teeth and jaws are clearly not designed to catch and rip up meat. Our teeth are designed for biting fruits and vegetables, just as our hands are designed for gathering them. We were designed to gather, not hunt.

➤ Our digestive tract is approximately twelve times as long as our body whilst that of the carnivore is only three times the length of it's body and is fairly straight. When a carnivore eats flesh and bone, the food moves through its system quickly, aided by a strong concentration of hydrochloric acid. When a human attempts to digest flesh foods, the process is very slow and laboured with the meat usually putrefying in the process.

➤ Large amounts of uric acid is produced from the diet containing meat. The consumption carnivorous animals have relatively larger kidneys to handle this burden whereas humans do not.

➤ Most of us could not tolerate meat in its raw form nor could we tolerate having to kill and butcher an animal ourselves without feeling ill.

➤ Meat is a second-hand source of vitamins, minerals and protein. Nearly all animals eaten by other animals are themselves herbivores. Vegetation is where the nutrition originally comes from.

➤ Nitrogen wastes from eating animal products create uric acid in large amounts. This overworks the kidneys, causing kidney disease and contributing to many complaints including rheumatic problems such as arthritis, gout and cataracts.

➤ The eating of meat leads to nutritional deficiencies. It has little calcium but plenty of phosphorus, which leaches calcium from the cells. High-level meat consumption also results in B6, niacin and magnesium deficiencies.

➤ The animal fats contain hormones, which can cause imbalances in our sexual/emotional lives and over stimulating certain organs.

➤ After the animal is killed, the cells continue functioning for a time, producing wastes. There is no blood circulation to carry these away, so the wastes remain in the tissues.

> Nearly all meat is eaten cooked, which greatly diminishes its value as a protein food. Cooking destroys amino acids, numerous vitamins and organic minerals. Cooked meat produces a high white blood cell count and may lead to leukaemia.

> Meat often contains residues of the various drugs that the animal was given before it was killed. These drugs include anti-biotics, hormones (linked with changes in sexual functions and appearance, pelvic and reproductive organ cancer, as well as sterilization in young people).

> Before being slaughtered, the animal is no doubt in a terrified state. This terror releases chemicals, which get passed into whoever eat the meat. This is not an energetic state I would chose to absorb into my body.

> When I watch meat eaters tucking into a plate of cooked flesh, I notice that they are rarely in a calm and peaceful state of mind. It hit home about ten years ago when I was observing a group of four men eating meat together in a café. Folk seem to become somewhat animalistic when they eat meat and this to me is another reason why I am vegetarian; I want to evolve and rid myself of these animalistic tendencies.

COMMERCIALLY PROCESSED MEAT IS EXCEPTIONALLY BAD FOR THE HEALTH

Some meat products are worse than others. Commercially processed meat (such as burgers and chicken nuggets) is far more dangerous than organically fed free range meat.

Mechanically reclaimed meat refers to the horrific process of blasting a carcass with powerful jets of air to obtain the last dregs of 'meat' from the unfortunate animal. This type of meat is sold in

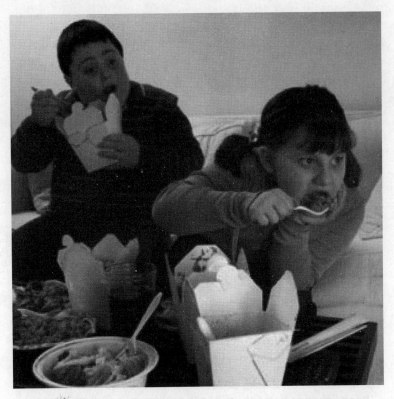

Fig. 5.4 These unfortunate young children can look forward to
any number of illnesses related to obesity and toxemia in
the coming years, thanks to their junk food lifestyle.

massive quantities all over the world and contains such delights as:

- Artificial colouring agents such as sodium sulphite, which restores the red colour and eliminates the foul smell of rotting flesh.
- Artificial flavours, including MSG.
- Preservatives like formaldehyde, alum, sodium chloride and sodium nitrite.

Fish is often not that much better...

Contrary to popular belief, fish consumption is also a poor dietary choice. Ocean fish pick up a lot of pollution, especially if they swim around the coastal areas (where human waste is pumped).

After being caught, fish are often sprayed with formaldehyde, whilst fresh water fish contains mercury, polychlorinated biphenyls (PCB's) and other industrial wastes that are poured into the waters.

Nor is cheese & pasteurised milk...

Pasteurised milk contains:

> ➢ Up to 59 hormones
>
> ➢ Up to 52 antibiotics
>
> ➢ Dozens of allergens
>
> ➢ Herbicides
>
> ➢ Pesticides
>
> ➢ Dioxins

All these are heavily concentrated during the cheese making process.

'In reality, cow's milk, especially processed cow's milk, has been linked to a variety of health problems, including: mucous production, haemoglobin loss, childhood diabetes, heart disease, atherosclerosis, arthritis, kidney stones, mood swings, depression, irritability, allergies...'

- Townsend Medical Letter, May, 1995

'Milk and milk products gave the highest correlation coefficient to heart disease, while sugar, animal proteins and animal fats came in second, third and fourth, respectively.'

- A Survey of Mortality Rates and Food Consumption Statistics of 24 countries, Medical Hypothesis, 7:907-918, 1981

'Rheumatoid arthritis is more severe than osteoarthritis, is most common in the hands and feet, and is characterised by swelling of joints. Since this type of joint pain can be a symptom of a food allergy, dietary change sometimes has a profound effect. Dairy products, the most common food allergen, are one likely candidate as a contributing causative factor.'

- Vegetarian and Vegan Nutrition,
George Eisman, M.A., M.Sc., R.D

Raw food

Largely overlooked by many 'fad' diet systems (as well as many macrobiotic, Chinese and Ayurvedic healthcare practitioners) is the importance of eating uncooked food regularly. Most people never take the time to consider why we feel the need to cook our food at high temperatures; yet the truth is clear that exposing food to fire destroys much of its goodness.

I know a few Japanese people who follow a Macrobiotic diet yet are not particularly healthy. They get the flu, have spots on their face and certainly don't appear to be in vibrant health. It turns out that they hard'y ever eat any raw food at all (and also don't feel that it is important to drink lots of pure water each day). I tell them 'You should eat more salad, more raw food and drink more water' but they just brush it off and continue with their deep fried tempeh and excessive rice intake. In Goa the locals sometimes laugh at me for suggesting that they should eat salad with their fish curry rice. They have an aversion to drinking water as well and they wonder why they grow old so quickly and suffer illness more than they should.

Exposing foods to temperatures over 118 degrees destroys many of its nutrients. It is only us, humans who indulge in this practice and it is also us, humans who are the sickest beings on earth. Whilst it is true that cooked food retains its nutrients, fats and vitamins etc, they exist in a way that the body cannot easily make use of it due to its altered molecular structure. Raw food is digested and assimilated in far easier way than cooked food primarily because the enzymes in the food are destroyed during the cooking process. Enzymes are what the body creates in order to make use of the nutrients.

Examples of foods which can be eaten in a 100% raw diet include:

> Minerals

Salads, lettuce, carrot leaves, kelp, grass juice.

> Fats

Nuts, seeds (sunflower, pumpkin, sesame), flaxseed (1-2 tbs. a day).

> Carbohydrate (simple sugars)

Fruit, especially bananas.

> Carbohydrate (complex)

Raw, (soaked overnight or slightly sprouted grains) hulled buckwheat, wheat, rye, oats, raw wheat germ, corn, yam.

> Complete protein foods (animal)

Eggs or fish can be immersed in boiling water for six seconds then eaten (can be marinated in lemon juice overnight to kill microbes), clams, oysters; dairy products, bee pollen.

> Vegetable proteins (which need to be complemented by grains or seeds or nuts to be complete proteins).

Legumes: mung beans or lentils or others (use 1/3 to 2/3 cup or 1.5 - 4 oz). Soak overnight or sprout.

Nuts or seeds: Sunflowers, pumpkin, or hulled sesame (1 to 3 oz.). These can be complemented with legumes (1 or 2 oz. legumes with 1 to 2 oz. nuts or seeds).

Additional foods that can be eaten raw include:

➢ Brewer's Yeast: will complement grains (1 tbs. maximum)

➢ Seaweed: kelp, dulse, others (1 tbs. to 1 oz. Maximum)

➢ Tubers: yam, potato, chestnuts

➢ Oil: Hempseed, coconut, flaxseed, virgin olive oil (1 to 4 tbs. per day)

➢ Herbs: fresh or dried basil, dill, parsley, garlic; young coconut

*1 fl. oz. = 30 ml

SAMPLE 100% RAW DIET MENU

Breakfast:

➢ Vegetable Juice (optional), (8 oz.) or a pint of hot water with a pinch of salt, a tablespoon of molasses syrup and a tablespoon of apple cider vinegar

➢ Mixed fruit salad (8 to 12 oz.)

➢ Sunflower seeds or almonds (1 to 2 oz.)

Lunch:

➢ Juice (optional), same as above

➢ Mixed salad (8 - 12 oz.), same as above with 1-2 tbs. of mung beans (soaked or sprouted) and 1 tbs. whole flaxseed ground

➢ 1 fruit (8 oz.)

➢ Seeds or nuts

Evening:

> ➤ Tossed salad (Romaine, cucumber, celery, pepper, tomato) and l-2 tbs of mung beans

> ➤ Grains (1 tbs. or more) of soaked, hulled buckwheat (sprouted or you may add soaked wheat, triticale, rye, or other) plus 1 tbs. of rice polishings

Snack (optional):

> ➤ Shredded raw yam and carrots, or up to two bananas

You may omit breakfast or lunch if you don't feel hungry or permanently, if one or two meals per day are desired.

Sprouting seeds, beans, grains, nuts and pulses

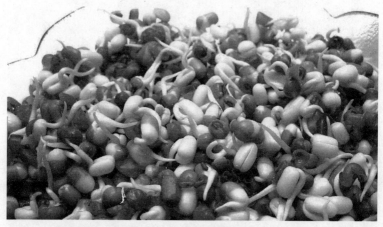

Fig. 5.5 Freshly sprouted organic mung beans.

One of the most powerful and inexpensive ways to obtain enormous amounts of vitamins, minerals, proteins and enzymes is to eat sprouts on a regular basis. Sprout eaters often say that they can 'feel' the goodness after eating them. Sprouted seeds, beans and grains aid digestion, build strong nerve tissue, bones and blood helping with anti-aging and over-coming disease. Enzymes help the digestive process to assimilate proteins, carbohydrates and fat. By 1930 only eighty different enzymes had been identified; today that figure has grown to four thousand.

PURE, NATURAL, ORGANIC AND VERY EASY TO CULTIVATE AT HOME

Depending on what is being sprouted and for how long, there is between ten and one hundred times more enzymes in sprouts than available in raw fruits and vegetables. Enzymes are extremely important in anti-aging and general healthcare because as we get older, our body generally loses the ability to produce digestive enzymes. Why? Because eating cooked, processed and denatured food has meant that our bodies have been forced to produce excessively concentrated enzymes for many years - just to break down the poor quality foods we have been feeding to ourselves. Our body's ability to make enzymes is not unlimited. If we lived on a completely organic, raw food diet, we would have all the nutrients (including enzymes) we need but in today's age, very few are willing or able to adopt a 100% raw/organic diet. Eating sprouts can rectify this problem easily.

TURBO CHARGE HEALTH BY HARNESSING THE POWER OF NATURE

Sprouts are truly a food for the future but by no means were they unknown to the ancients. Five thousand years ago, Chinese nobles were using them for healing and rejuvenation and more recently, during WW2 in the United States, scientists advised the president that sprouts were the cheapest and best alternative source of protein to meat. Unlike in meat, sprouts are a complete protein; exactly as nature intended.

When examining what happens during germination it looks like a vitamin factory. Below are nutritional comparisons:

> Alfalfa sprouts have more chlorophyll than spinach, kale, cabbage or parsley. Alfalfa, sunflower, clover and radish sprouts are all 4% protein whereas spinach is only 3%, Romaine lettuce is1.5% and Iceberg lettuce is 0.8%, and milk is 3.3%.

> Meat is 19% and eggs are 13% protein (and 11% fat) whereas Soybean sprouts have 28% protein, and lentil and pea sprouts are 26%. Soybean sprouts have twice the protein of eggs and only 1/10 of the fat.

> Grain and nut sprouts, such as wheat and sunflower, are rich in fats. While fats in flour and wheat germ have a reputation for going rancid quickly (stores should refrigerate them), fats in sprouts last for weeks.

> The valuable wheat germ oil in wheat sprouts is broken down into its essential fatty acid fractions (over 50% of which is Omega 6.).

> While sunflower oil is a fine source of omega 6, germination of the sunflower sprout changes the fatty acids into an easily digestible, water soluble form saving our body the trouble of breaking it down whilst simultaneously protecting us against the perils of rancidity.

> Radish sprouts have 29 times more Vitamin C and 4 times more Vitamin A than milk, and 39 times more provitamin than mature radishes.

There have been many other observations and studies into sprouts, which back-up the fact that they are well worth growing and consuming. Here are some of the sprouts to try. Out of these, I like to sprout hemp seeds, mung beans and alfalfa seeds the best.

The following table shows some of the more popular sprouts and their health benefits:

Alfalfa	Alfalfa is abundant in vital nutrients. If we were forced to live solely on one type of food our choice should probably be alfalfa! It's rich in vitamins A, B complex, C, E and K; it's rich in calcium, magnesium, potassium, iron, selenium and zinc and it cleanses the blood and the liver.
Chickpeas	Chickpeas are 25% by weight protein and are rich in fatty acids, carbohydrates and fibre. These are high in vitamins A and C and are rich in calcium, magnesium and potassium. Because they help build red blood cells these are good for anaemia and they help fight cancer and build muscle tissue. The seeds of chickpeas contain trypsin inhibitors, which interfere with protein digestion. Although cooking reduces these inhibitors, these can still be difficult to digest even when cooked and often cause gas and bloating. However, when sprouted the active enzymes neutralise the trypsin inhibitors so these can usually be eaten raw without digestive discomfort.
Fenugreek	This easy to grow sprout is rich in iron, phosphorous and potassium and is high in vitamins A and C. It can be mixed with milder sprouts such as alfalfa and clover. It cleanses the body of toxins, helps stabilise blood sugar and helps with intestinal problems such as IBS, colon cancer and diverticulitis. It has a soothing mucilaginous gel which coats and protects all the veins and organs of the body. In a Harvard University study, 58% of a group of diabetics given fenugreek either came off insulin completely or reduced their dosage dramatically.

Hemp	This is one of the most nutritionally complete foods on the planet (See the Super foods section: Hempseed oil). It contains all 8 essential amino acids in a favourable ratio and is 36% protein. It contains omega 9 and the EFAs omega 3 & 6 (1:3 omega 3:omega 6). It's also the highest natural source of GLA (a type of super omega 6 that has strong anti-inflammatory properties). It also contains about 26 different minerals, has significant quantities of lecithin and is good for all things related to the heart and the head. When you sprout the hemp seed, the nutrients multiply around 20 times. The seeds from some suppliers don't sprout, perhaps because they've been irradiated.
Lentils	There are various types of lentils, which can be mixed together. They're an excellent source of vitamin C, although in their dormant state they have virtually no vitamin C at all. They're also rich in iron and amino acids. They taste chalky on account of their bone building minerals.
Mung	Mung beans are a very good source of protein, vitamin C, iron, potassium and zinc. They are extremely digestible and help prevent prostate cancer, premature greying of the hair and balding. When grown commercially, they are kept under pressure and grown in darkness to make them long and succulent. So, two days after they have begun to sprout put a heavy weight on them (try sprouting them in a cafeteria with the lid pressed down!) and put them in darkness (wrap in a black

	bin liner). This will encourage the sprouts to produce ethylene gas thus forcing them to grow faster and whiter.
Sunflower	Sunflower is a complete protein and has all of the 8 essential amino acids. In fact, it has a perfect balance of protein and fats. It builds all tissue, all muscle, all cartilage and all myelin. Like buckwheat you can either eat it as sprouted seeds (use the silver hulled seeds) or grow it as sunflower greens. It is rich in different essential minerals constituents as it provides potassium, for the nervous system, magnesium for muscle, tissue, brain and lungs and has lots of phosphorous and calcium also.

Sprouting is easy and it doesn't require any soil or fertiliser. In only 2-7 days, the nutritional content of the seed etc increases from 25% to 4,000%.

'Sproutman' (Alias: Steve Meyerowitz) has been actively promoting sprouts since the 1970's. He says:

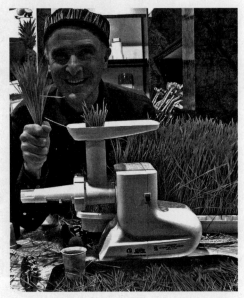

Fig. 5.6 Sproutman (Alias: Steve Meyerowitz)

'Sprouts are baby plants in their prime. They have a greater concentration of proteins, vitamins and minerals, enzymes, RNA, DNA, bio-flavinoids, T-cells etc than any other point in the plants life even when compared with the mature vegetable!'

The easiest method is to use a commercial sprouting device. Other ways make use of jars, trays or bags. Small seeds and seeds which develop leaves (alfalfa, broccoli, clover, radish) do well in trays, jars or bags whereas larger seeds (mung and chickpeas) do well in jars or bags, but not in trays.

HOW TO SPROUT

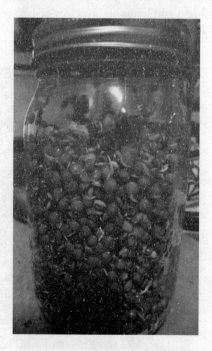

Fig. 5.7 (a) A simple sprouting jar.

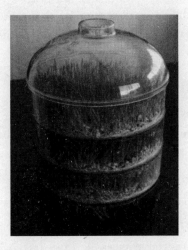

Fig. 5.7 (b) Sprouting trays for large scale production.

Perhaps the simplest way to grow sprouts at home is to soak them in a cup of water for 24 hours, drain them and then place them in a desert bowl. Cover the desert bowl with a plate and leave to stand. Pour water into the bowl twice per day and then drain it off by turning the bowl upside down over the sink (remember to hold the sieve tightly in place). In no time at all ,you will have a bowl brimming full of vibrant sprouts!

Put seeds in a jar and soak overnight in water (as pure as possible). Large seeds (e.g. chickpeas) need lots of water. If the seeds have absorbed all the water add some more and soak for longer, making sure you use more next time. Rinse twice a day (3 times if the weather is hot) by putting under the cold tap and washing thoroughly so that any foam comes out of the jar. After each rinse drain well at an angle of 45 degrees.

No one who can afford to eat junk food can truthfully say they can't afford to eat healthily. Simply buy a bag of seeds/grains and sprout them. Only a small portion of these sprouts is needed to obtain optimum nutrition and they are easy to incorporate as a valuable addition to any diet.

HEALTHY SPROUT RECIPE IDEAS

- ➢ Add to tossed salads
- ➢ Eat them fresh and uncooked in a sprout salad
- ➢ Try in sandwiches and wraps
- ➢ On top of toast, olive-hempseed oil and spirulina
- ➢ Stir-fry with other vegetables
- ➢ Blend into fruit shakes or juices
- ➢ Blend with vegetable juices
- ➢ Grind up and use in sandwich spreads
- ➢ Put on top of your grilled cheese sandwiches
- ➢ Stir into soups or stews when serving
- ➢ Combine in rice dishes
- ➢ Use sprouted chickpeas (or hemp seeds) for raw humus recipies
- ➢ Saute with onions
- ➢ Puree with peas or beans
- ➢ Add to baked beans
- ➢ Steam and serve with butter

Juicing

Juicing fruits and vegetables with a home juicer is an excellent way to take in large amounts of natural goodness without having to eat regular large meals. For instance, one kilogram of organic carrots can be juiced into about 400ml of tasty juice, giving the body a large dose of all the vitamins and minerals that carrot contains, particularly vitamin A.

Most of the fibre is removed during the juicing process, meaning that drinking juices puts very little strain on the digestive system and will often give healthy energy boost.

Below is a list of various foods that can be juiced:

> Alfalfa sprouts
> Apple
> Beetroot
> Brocolli
> Carrot
> Celery
> Cherry (Cherries)
> Cucumber
> Fennel

- ➢ Garlic
- ➢ Ginger
- ➢ GrapeFruit
- ➢ Grapes
- ➢ Kiwi Fruit
- ➢ Lemon
- ➢ Lettuce
- ➢ Lime
- ➢ Melon
- ➢ Mung bean sprouts
- ➢ Nectarine
- ➢ Noni
- ➢ Orange
- ➢ Parsnip
- ➢ Peach
- ➢ Pear
- ➢ Pepper
- ➢ Pineapple
- ➢ Plum
- ➢ Pomegranate
- ➢ Radish
- ➢ Strawberry
- ➢ Tomato
- ➢ Watermelon
- ➢ Wheat grass

Using a spinning blades blender for making juice will damage its delicate structure and render it nutritionally inferior. The grinding/pressing models are far superior (see the Superfoods: Wheatgrass section of this chapter for information about juicing devices).

Acid / alkaline balance

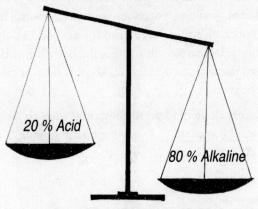

Fig. 5.8] Acid Alkaline Balance

One of the simplest ways to understand why so many of us are falling sick and not attaining the high levels of health, we are easily capable of is to realise that the vast majority of us are way too acidic in our bodies. In my experience, most people in the world are falling way short of the optimum 80 / 20 alkaline-acid balance. In short, as a species we've developed an unhealthy attraction to acid-forming foods.

An acidic bodily environment gives rise to an internal environment conducive to disease, as opposed to a pH-balanced environment which allows normal body function necessary for the body to resist disease. When excess acids must be neutralized our alkaline reserves are depleted leaving the body in a weakened condition.

The pH (the potential of hydrogen) is a measure of the acidity or alkalinity of a solution. It is measured on a scale of 0 to 14; the lower the pH the more acidic the solution, the higher the pH the more alkaline the solution.

This is not referring to stomach acid or the pH of the stomach. It refers to the pH of the body's fluids and tissues.

The condition of acidity forces the body to borrow minerals (such as calcium, sodium, potassium and magnesium) from vital organs and bones to buffer (neutralize) the acid and safely remove it from the body. Because of this strain, the body can suffer severe and prolonged damage due to high acidity; a condition that may go undetected for years.

Mild acidosis alone can lead to conditions such as:

➢ Cardiovascular damage (including the constriction of blood vessels and the reduction of oxygen)

➢ Weight gain

➢ Diabetes

➢ Bladder and kidney conditions

➢ Immune deficiency

➢ Acceleration of free radical damage (possibly contributing to cancerous mutations)

➢ Hormone concerns

➢ Premature aging

> Osteoporosis; weak, brittle bones, hip fractures and bone spurs
> Joint pain, aching muscles and lactic acid build-up
> Low energy and chronic fatigue
> Slow digestion and elimination
> Yeast/fungal overgrowth

A food's acid or alkaline-forming tendency in the body is not connected with the actual pH of the food itself. For example, lemons are very acidic; however they create alkalinity after digestion and assimilation. Likewise, meat will test alkaline before digestion but it leaves very acidic residue in the body and so, like nearly all animal products.

BALANCED MEAL PLANNING

Alkaline forming foods (80% of the daily diet should contain these foods):

> All vegetables (except dried beans, lentils, asparagus tips, and garbanzos).
> All fresh fruits (except cranberries, plums, olives, prunes, and blueberries) (Preserves and canned fruits are usually acid-forming).
> Almonds, chestnuts, Brazil nuts, and hazelnuts.

Acid forming foods (20 % of the daily diet should contain these foods):

> All grains, cereals, and bakery products except for soybeans.
> All dairy except buttermilk, yoghurt, raw milk and whey.
> Peanuts, pecans, and walnuts.

A few food combinations to avoid:

Certain food combinations are difficult to digest and may cause problems in the digestive system. Here is a brief list of food combinations to avoid:

> Two or more carbohydrates at the same meal
> Sugary foods and starchy foods
> Milk and citrus fruit / juice
> Cereals and citrus fruit / juice
> Large quantities of starchy foods with meat or cheese
> Coffee with milk or cream
> Raw apples with other foods

ALKALINE	ACID
ALKALIZING VEGETABLES	**ACIDIFYING VEGETABLES**
Alfalfa	Corn
Barley grass	Lentils
Beets	Olives
Beet greens	Winter squash
Broccoli	
Cabbage	**ACIDIFYING FRUITS**
Carrot	
Cauliflower	Blueberries

Celery

Chard greens

Chlorella

Collard greens

Cucumber

Dandelions

Edible flowers

Eggplant

Fermented veggies

Garlic

Green beans

Green peas

Kale

Kohlrabi

Lettuce

Mushrooms

Mustard greens

Nightshade veggies

Onions

Parsnips

Peas

Peppers

Pumpkin

Radishes

Canned or glazed fruits

Cranberries

Currants

Plums

Prunes

ACIDIFYING GRAINS, GRAIN PRODUCTS

Amaranth

Barley

Bran, wheat

Bran, oat

Corn

Cornstarch

Hemp seed flour

Kamut

Oats (rolled)

Oatmeal

Quinoa

Rice (all)

Rice cakes

Rye

Spelt

Rutabaga

Sea vegetables

Spinach, green

Spirulina

Sprouts

Sweet potatoes

Tomatoes

Watercress

Wheat grass

Wild greens

ALKALIZING
ORIENTAL VEGETABLES

Maitake

Daikon

Dandelion root

Shitake

Kombu

Reishi

Nori

Umeboshi

Wakame

Wheat

Wheat germ

Noodles

Macaroni

Spaghetti

Bread

Crackers, soda

Flour, white

Flour, wheat

ACIDIFYING
BEANS & LEGUMES

Black beans

Chick peas

Green peas

Kidney beans

Lentils

Pinto beans

Red beans

Soy beans

Soy milk

White beans

Rice Milk

Almond Milk

ALKALIZING FRUITS	ACIDIFYING DAIRY
Apple	Butter
Apricot	Cheese
Avocado	Cheese, processed
Banana (high glycemic)	Ice Cream
Berries	Ice Milk
Blackberries	
Cantaloupe	**ACIDIFYING NUTS & BUTTERS**
Cherries, sour	Cashews
Coconut, fresh	Legumes
Currants	Peanuts
Dates, dried	Peanut butter
Figs, dried	Pecans
Grapes	Tahini
Grapefruit	Walnuts
Honeydew melon	
Lemon	**ACIDIFYING ANIMAL PROTEIN**
Lime	Bacon
Muskmelons	Beef
Nectarine	Carp
Orange	Clams
Peach	Cod
Pear	

Pineapple	Corned beef
Raisins	Fish
Raspberries	Haddock
Rhubarb	Lamb
Strawberries	Lobster
Tangerine	Mussels
Tomato	Organ meats
Tropical fruits	Oyster
Umeboshi plums	Pike
Watermelon	Pork
	Rabbit
ALKALIZING PROTEIN	Salmon
Almonds	Sardines
Chestnuts	Sausage
Millet	Scallops
Tempeh (fermented)	Shrimp
Tofu (fermented)	Scallops
Whey protein powder	Shellfish
	Tuna
	Turkey
ALKALIZING SWEETENERS	Veal
Stevia	Venison

ALKALIZING SPICES & SEASONINGS	ACIDIFYING FATS & OILS
Cinnamon	Avacado oil
Curry	Butter
Ginger	Canola oil
Mustard	Corn oil
Chilli pepper	Hemp Seed oil
Sea salt	Flax oil
Miso	Lard
Tamari	Olive oil
All herbs	Safflower oil
	Sesame oil
ALKALIZING OTHER	Sunflower oil
Apple cider vinegar	
Bee pollen	**ACIDIFYING SWEETENERS**
Lecithin granules	Carob
Molasses, blackstrap	Sugar
Probiotic cultures	Corn syrup
Soured dairy products	
Green juices	**ACIDIFYING ALCOHOL**
Veggie juices	
Fresh fruit juice	Beer
Mineral water	Spirits
Alkaline antioxidant water	Wine

ALKALIZING MINERALS	**ACIDIFYING OTHER FOODS**
Cesium: pH 14	Catsup
Potassium: pH 14	Cocoa
Sodium: pH 14	Coffee
Calcium: pH 12	Vinegar
Magnesium: pH 9	Mustard
	Pepper
Although it might seem that citrus fruits would have an acidifying effect on the body, the citric acid they contain actually has an alkalizing effect in the bodily system.	Soft drinks
	ACIDIFYING DRUGS & CHEMICALS
	Aspirin
	Chemicals
	Drugs, medicinal
	Drugs, psychedelic
	Pesticides
	Herbicides
	Tobacco
	ACIDIFYING JUNK FOOD
	Coca-Cola: pH 2
	Beer: pH 2.5
	Coffee: pH 4

There are several versions of the acidic and alkaline food chart to be found in different books and on the Internet.

The following foods are sometimes attributed to the acidic side of the chart and sometimes to the alkaline side.

Asparagus, Brazil nuts, Brussels sprouts, buckwheat, chicken, corn, cottage cheese, eggs, flax seeds, green tea, herbal tea, honey, kombucha, lima beans, maple syrup, milk, nuts, potatoes, pumpkin seeds, sauerkraut, soy products, sprouted seeds, squashes, sunflower seeds.

Very alkaline:

Lemons, watermelon, soaked figs, mango, melons, baking soda.

Very acidic:

Artificial sweeteners, beef, beer, breads, brown sugar, carbonated soft drinks, c(refined), chocolate, cigarettes / tobacco, coffee, custard (with white sugar), drugs generally, fish, flour (white wheat), fruit Juices with sugar, jams, jellies, lamb, liquor, maple syrup (processed), pasta (white), pastries and cakes from white flour, pickles (commercial), pork, poultry, seafood, sugar (white), table salt (refined and iodized), tea (black), white bread, white vinegar (processed), whole wheat foods, wine, yoghurt (sweetened).

ACID / ALKALINE HEALTH TIPS

> ➤ Chew food until saliva breaks it down properly.
> ➤ Drink minimal fluids with your meals.
> ➤ Avoid food with pesticides and preservatives.
> ➤ Avoid large meals and cooked food.
> ➤ Eat salads regularly.
> ➤ Drink a glass of water with 1/2 teaspoon of baking soda stirred into it to lower hyper-acidity in the body.

CHECKING ACID / ALKALINE LEVELS

It is simple to monitor your pH checking both urine and saliva with test strips. These strips are available from good pharmacies and via the Internet.

The lower the reading, the more acidic your body is and the more difficult it is for it to repair itself because it is in a degenerative state. In most cases, people with cancer and other serious health problems are very acidic. It is amazing at how terribly acid-forming soda, coffee, tea and beer are if you check them with litmus paper. Likewise check the worst and best foods with litmus paper also so as to understand more how important it is to eat properly.

How to determine your body pH value

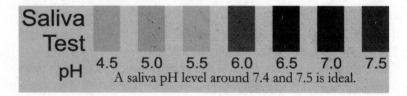

A saliva pH level around 7.4 and 7.5 is ideal.

Firstly, clean your hands so they don't influence the test when you touch the paper. Perform the colour chart test at least two hours after any food has been eaten. Apply saliva to the litmus paper strip for a few seconds and then wait for twenty seconds.

The litmus paper will change colour to indicate your body's pH measurement. Compare it to the pH colour chart below. (The dry colour of a pH strip can vary somewhat. However, when submerged in saliva, it will accurately reflect the pH level.)

The acidity and the alkalinity in the body is determined by the pH (hydrogen potential) scale. Water has a pH of 7.0 and is considered neutral; neither acidic or alkaline. The ideal bodily pH value is 7.4

or 7.5. The body is considered acidic if below 7.0, and alkaline if above 7.8.

The pH of different parts of the body is of crucial importance.

The mouth should be alkaline (greater than 7.0) for salivary enzymes to function.

The stomach should be acidic (less than 6.3) to digest protein properly.

The small intestine should be alkaline for the pancreatic enzymes to work.

The large intestine should be a little acidic to maintain proper bowel flora. Other parts of the body have different pH values.

Super foods

The term 'super food' refers to those foods that have a particularly beneficial affect on health, included below are some of the finest super foods on the planet.

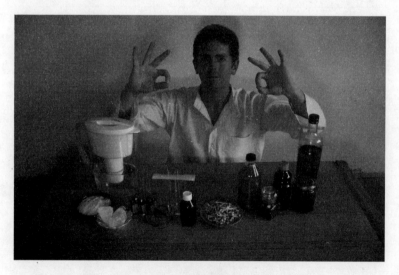

Fig. 5.9 The author with filtered water, Himalayan crystal salt, home made colloidal silver, sprouted mung beans, apple cider vinegar, powdered spirulina, hemp seed oil, molasses syrup and olive oil

APPLE CIDER VINEGAR

Apples are a powerful and highly nutritional food. Apple cider vinegar is liquid made from fermented apples and only a teaspoon or two is needed each day to reap a wide variety of health benefits.

The apple cider vinegar is loaded with the life-building mineral potassium. The potassium is to the soft tissue what calcium is to the bones and hard tissue and it is the key mineral in that it causes the soft tissue of life forms (including plants) to grow. Potassium deficiency is a serious problem in the modern world and leads to such health problems as:

- Loose, wrinkled skin
- Dry, greying and balding hair/scalp
- Impediment of physical growth
- Weakened eyesight
- Itchy, sore, dry eyes
- Memory loss

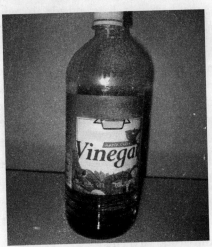

Fig. 5.10 Apple Cider Vinegar

> Lethargy
> Nervousness
> Depression
> Headaches
> Dizziness
> Cold hand and feet

The human body is constantly regenerating itself:

> Every 90 days a new bloodstream is created
> Every 11 months a new set of body cells are created
> Every 7 years we have an entirely new set of bones and hard tissues

This generally happens, thanks to our food, drink and air intake. Back in 1914, Dr. Alexis Carrel began an experiment by which he kept the cells of an embryo chicken heart functioning for thirty years by daily monitoring of its nutrition, cleansing and elimination. Considering the normal life span of a chicken only seven or eight years, it seems that he may well have made an important discovery; that it is not age which kills a man but rather man kills himself with incorrect diet and lifestyle habits.

In the same way, vinegar removes grime from windows, in apple cider vinegar, potassium enters into clogged, caked arteries and cleans them out. If the arteries are clogged with toxic poisons we can't think properly; in fact senility is often the result of blocked arteries.

Apple cider vinegar is extremely broad spectrum in its various applications (it has a lot of uses). These include:

> Headaches
> Weight gain / loss
> Sore throat and laryngitis
> Skin care

> Scalp care
> Corns, calluses and warts
> Joint pain

Apple cider vinegar can be mixed into a drink or used with oil on a salad. Generally one tablespoon mixed with hot water and sweetened with molasses syrup or honey is taken once or twice per day is recommended.

BLACKSTRAP MOLASSES SYRUP

Blackstrap molasses is made from the third boiling of the sugar syrup and is therefore, the concentrated by-product left over after the

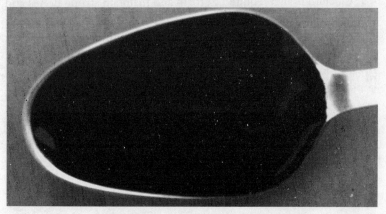

Fig. 5.11 Blackstrap Molasses Syrup

sugar's sucrose has been crystallized. Unlike other sweeteners such as refined sugar or corn syrup, molasses contains a large amount of important minerals. Some of these minerals include:

> Iron
> Calcium
> Copper
> Manganese

> ➢ Potassium
> ➢ Magnesium

Iron is particularly important for pregnant women who are often at risk from iron deficiency. Iron is a key constituent of haemoglobin (which transports oxygen from the lungs to all body cells) and is also part of key enzyme systems for energy production and metabolism.

Calcium is one of the most important minerals as it is involved in a variety of physiological activities essential to life. These include the ability of the heart and other muscles to contract, blood clotting, the conduction of nerve impulses to and from the brain, regulation of enzyme activity, and cell membrane function.

Calcium is also required to form and maintain strong bones and teeth and to help prevent the loss of bone that can occur during menopause and as a result of rheumatoid arthritis. Calcium binds to toxins and removes them from the colon, thus reducing the risk of auto-intoxication/toxemia. Calcium is also is involved in nerve conduction.

Copper is an essential component of many enzymes and plays a role in physiological processes such as for the elimination of free radicals, development of bone and connective tissue, and the production of melanin (a skin and hair pigment).

Many health problems can be caused by copper deficiency, such as:

> ➢ Anemia
> ➢ Ruptured blood vessels
> ➢ Osteoporosis
> ➢ Joint pain / rheumatoid arthritis
> ➢ Brain disturbances
> ➢ Imbalanced LDL and HDL cholesterol levels
> ➢ Irregular heartbeat
> ➢ Increased susceptibility to infections

Manganese is a trace mineral that helps produce energy from protein and carbohydrates. It is also involved in the synthesis of fatty acids (which are important for a healthy nervous system).

Manganese is also an important component of the antioxidant enzyme named superoxide dismutase, which is found inside the body's of mitochondria (the oxygen-based energy factories inside most of our cells). Inside the mitochondria, it serves to protect against damage from the free radicals produced during energy production.

Potassium is needed for muscle contraction and nerve transmission. It is also involved in carbohydrate storage for use by muscles as fuel as well as in maintaining the body's proper electrolyte and acid / alkaline balance. Potassium deficiency causes a decrease in glycogen (the fuel used by exercising muscles) levels.

Magnesium is calcium's major balancing mineral and like calcium, it is necessary for healthy teeth, bones and energy production. Symptoms of magnesium deficiency include:

➢ High blood pressure

➢ Muscle spasms (including heart and bronchiole spasms)

➢ Migraines

➢ Muscle cramps

➢ Tension

➢ Soreness

➢ Fatigue

Avoid processed or 'sulphured' molasses syrup and try to find an organic variety if possible. Most large supermarkets and health food shops supply molasses at a cheap price.

1-2 tablespoons per day is a recommended adult dose. I like to mix a pint of hot water with molasses, apple cider vinegar and salt (see the Hot water & salt based elixirs section of the Salt chapter).

COCONUT WATER & OIL

Coconuts have been used for centuries in tropical areas of the world as a vital source of food for health and general well being. Recent research verifies traditional beliefs that the coconut palm is a 'Tree

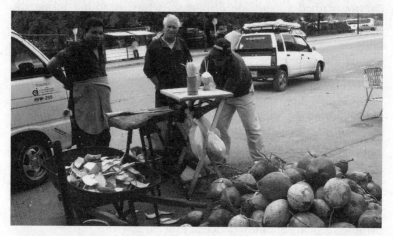

Fig. 5.12 Fresh coconut water being sold by the roadside in India

of Life'. Coconut water and virgin coconut oil are indeed a powerful and abundant super food.

Tender coconut water contains a wealth of goodness, including:

- Magnesium
- Calcium
- Phosphorus
- Potassium
- Iron
- Sodium
- Ascorbic Acid (C)
- Thiamin (B1)

➤ Riboflavin (B2)
➤ Niacin (B3)
➤ Panththenic Acid (B5)
➤ Pyridoxine (B6)

All the goodness is contained in a pure, liquid form and thus is easy for the body to assimilate.

Health benefits

➤ Improves kidney, liver and heart functions
➤ Enhances the urinary tract elimination process
➤ Aids the elimination of toxins
➤ Electrolytes in coconut water re-balance the body's fluid balance
➤ Promoting weight loss when and if you need it
➤ Antibacterial, antimicrobial and antiprotozoal properties
➤ Provides the organism with healthy nutrients and enhances the body's vitality
➤ The balanced proportion of potassium, calcium, magnesium and sodium foster a speedy revitalisation and re-hydration
➤ Enhances concentration
➤ Provides an immediate energy source
➤ Prevents headaches by providing the body with all the necessary replenishing fluids
➤ Impacts positively on the electrolyte level content in the body

The virgin coconut oil is unique in its structural make-up and its saturated fat is highly beneficial for the human body. Included in this 92% saturated fat content is the highest source of saturated medium chain triglycerides (MCT's) of any naturally occurring vegan food source (62%). Furthermore, around 50% of these MCT's are made up of lauric acid, the most important essential fatty acid in building and maintaining the body's immune system.

Apart from coconut oil, the only other source of lauric acid found in such high concentrations is in mother's milk.

One negative study, conducted over forty years ago, has tarnished the reputation of coconut oil as part of a healthy diet. The oil that was used in this study was hydrogenated, yet the myth of coconut oil being dangerous to the health persists in many people's minds (like the negative studies using table salt in place of real salt).

'Never before in the history of man is it so important to emphasize the value of Lauric Oils. The medium chain fats in coconut oil are similar to fats in mother's milk and have similar nutriceutical effects.'

- Jon J. Kabara, PhD, Professor Emeritus,
Michigan State University

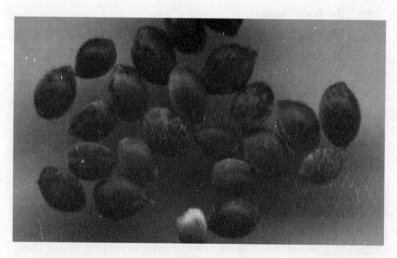

Fig. 5.13 Hempseeds

HEMPSEED OIL

Widely believed to be the most balanced and nutritious oil available; hempseed oil serves as both food and medicine for a wide variety of health complaints. It is made from the cold pressed hemp seed, has a pleasant nutty taste and contains a plethora of goodness, including:

> Phosphorus

> Potassium

> Magnesium

> Sulphur

> Calcium

> Iron

> zinc.

> Carotene

> Protein

> Fibre

> Antioxidants (Vitamin E)

> Phytosterols

> Phospholipids

> Chlorophyll

> Essential fatty acids (EFA's)

We need essential fatty acids in our diet more than any other vitamin and research is linking EFA deficiencies with a variety of degenerative diseases including:

> Cardiovascular disease

> Cancer

> Diabetes

> Skin conditions

> Multiple Sclerosis

> PMS

> ➤ Heart problems
> ➤ Behavioural problems
> ➤ Poor wound healing
> ➤ Joint pain
> ➤ Glandular atrophy
> ➤ Weakened immunity
> ➤ Sterility in males

The hemp seed has both a high content of easy digestible, complete protein and a rich endowment of oil; this combination provides the most favourable ratio of Essential Fatty Acids (EFAs) required for proper human nutrition.

Our bodies use EFAs to:

> ➤ Construct membranes
> ➤ Create electrical potentials
> ➤ Move electric currents throughout the body

The chemical reactions on which life depends require a one-way movement of energy through molecules. EFAs play an important role in this function for the following reasons:

> ➤ Facilitates the recovery of fatigued muscles after exercise.
> ➤ Precursors of prostaglandins, a hormone-like substance that regulate cell functions in all tissues.
> ➤ Found around the hereditary material in our chromosomes, where they may play a part in maintaining chromosome stability and may have functions in starting and stopping gene expression.
> ➤ Helps our immune system resist and fight infections and prevent allergies from developing.
> ➤ Necessary for the development of brain and nerve cells and for healthy liver function

The following chart shows a comparison of EFA content for various different oils:

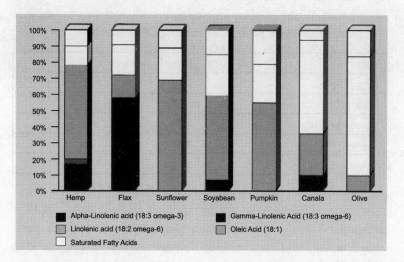

Hempseed oil costs around £20-25 / litre and is available from decent health food shops. Try to find oil that is fresh, stored in a fridge and in a tinted glass bottle. Also aim to find organic, cold pressed hempseed oil.

Hempseed oil is very delicate and should never be exposed to high temperatures. Because of its delicious taste, it can be used in a number of different ways, including:

➤ Use as part of a salad dressing

➤ Mix with fruit/vegetable juices

➤ Pour on any meal

➤ Pour on toast

➤ Simply take a small sip from the bottle

➤ Recommended adult dose is 1-4 tablespoons per day.

SPIRULINA

Spirulina contains eighteen of the twenty-two amino acids that the body needs. When compared with foods such as pulses and eggs, it has many times more protein, as shown in the table below:

Food	Protein content
Egg (10g)	1.1g
Milk (10g)	0.32g
Soyabean (10g)	3.7g
Pulses (10g)	1.8g
Spirulina	6.6g

Many people are saying that spirulina is indeed the most powerful and balanced source of nutrition on this planet. In 1974 in United Nation – World Health Organization (WHO) declared spirulina as 'The Best Food for Tomorrow'. NASA declared that 1Kg. of spirulina contains as much nutrition as 1000 Kg. of assorted vegetables.

Health benefits

> It has more beta-carotene (pro-vitamin A), iron and vitamin B12 than any other food.

> Abundant in trace elements, minerals, chlorophyll and enzymes (like zinc, calcium, magnesium, selenium, iron and phosphorus).

> Rich source of anti oxidants and beta-carotene to reduce chronic deficient disease.

> It is phyto-protein without the fat and cholesterol present in meat.

> A complete nutrient for malnourished children.

> Iron bioavailability that helps building blood cells.

> Builds strong immune system.

> Helps in kidney and liver function and reduce mercury, drugs, and chemical pollutant intake.

> Builds healthy lactobacillus.

> Helps in enhancing pancreas function which produces insulin to maintain blood sugar in the body.

According to Kelly Moorhead and Helen Morgan in their book 'Spirulina, Nature's Superfood', Spirulina is a rich source of:

> Vitamins

> Minerals

> Enzymes

> RNA

> DNA

> Sulfolipids

> Glycogen

> Other potentially important trace elements and nutrients

The following chart gives a nutritional profile of 100g of Spirulina:

Mositure	7g
Ash	9g
Protein	71g
Crude fibre	0.9g
Xanthophylls	180mg
Carotene	190mg
Chlorophyll	760mg
Vitamins	
Thiamine (B1)	5.5mg

Riboflavin (B2)	4.0mg
Nicotinic acid (B3)	0.3mg
Inositol (amino acid)	35mg
Pyridoxide (B6)	0.3mg
Cyano cobalamine (B12)	0.2mg
Tocopherol (Vitamin E)	19mg
Biotin (Vitamin H)	0.04g
GLA (Vitamin F)	1.3g
Minerals	
Calcium	132mg
Phosphorus	894mg
Iron	58mg
Zinc	3.9mg

When I last visited Sai Baba's ashram in Puttarparti, India (2005), I heard that the Sathya Sai General Hospital was giving fresh, locally

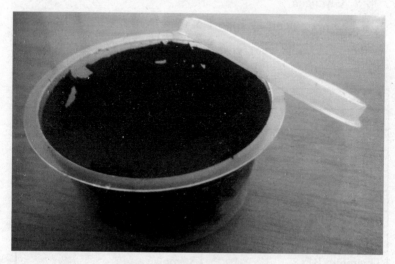

Fig. 5.14 Spirulina Paste

grown Spirulina to patients. I visited the small farm and found that the profits made from this cottage industry went towards taking care of the sick animals in the area. The project was run by a Dutch lady and a couple of local workers. I found out that she was also selling organic vegetables, colloidal silver and Himalayan rock salt (which she also used in the water in which the spirulina was grown).

The micro algae were grown in a large circular concrete pond with netting over the top and a mechanical arm that slowly moves through the water. When I last looked at www.youtube.com I found a few interesting videos about spirulina farming.

The spirulina powder is superior to the tablets as it has not been through the same mechanical processes, it also gives good value for your money – Retailing in the UK for approximately £40 for 500g. It has a pleasant taste and can be mixed with various foods, such as salads, spirulina/hempseed oil on toast being a particularly healthy and tasty snack.

WHEATGRASS JUICE

The wheat grass is the green, growing and processing plant that will eventually become a shaft of wheat and produces grain. After only one week in the sun, wheat grass reaches six to nine inches and can be cut and juiced. The deep green juice is abundant with vitamins, minerals, enzymes, chlorophyll and vital life energy. It is intensely concentrated and benefits can be quickly noticed with as little as one small gulp per day.

The main component in wheat grass is chlorophyll. That alone would be enough to bring great benefit however in its natural state, with appropriate proportion it is a powerful nutrient. Researcher Dr. Hans Fischer and his associates won the Nobel Prize for their work investigating the properties of red blood cells. One of the key points of the research found that chlorophyll and haemoglobin, the oxygen-binding substance in red blood cells, (RBC) were nearly identical molecules, chlorophyll is the 'blood' of plants.

Other researchers found that injections of chlorophyll caused an increase in haemoglobin levels and regeneration of red blood

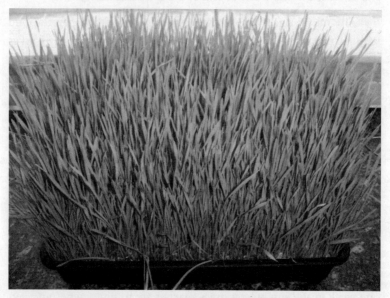

Fig. 5.15 A tray of eight-day-old Wheatgrass.

cells over 50% higher than usual. When erythropoiesis, (the forming of red blood cells) is higher, oxygenation is higher and the system in general benefits in a variety of ways.

The amino acid content of wheatgrass juice (Anne Quigmore, 1989).

Abensic	Anti cancer agent
Alanine	Blood builder
Arginine	Seminal fluid
Aspartic acid	Energy
Glutamic acid	Mental alertness
Glycine	Energy
Histidine	Hearing and nerve function
Isoleucine	Growth in infants
Loucine	Energy and nerve stimulation
Lysine	Anti aging
Methionine	Kidney and liver cleanser
Phenylaianine	Thyroid function
Proline	Glutamic acid absorption
Serine	Brain stimulation
Threonine	Digestion and assimilation
Tryptophane	Skin and hair growth
Valine	Brain muscle coordination

The enzyme content of Wheatgrass juice (Steve Meyerowitz, 1998)

Amylase	Facilitates starch digestion
Cytochrome Oxidase	Anti oxidant
Lipase	A fat splitting enzyme
Protease	Assists in protein digestion
Soperoxide Dismutase (SOD)	Found in all body cells and is known for its ability to lessen the effect of radiation and slow cellular aging
Transhydrogenase	Keeps heart muscle toned

Health benefits

- ➤ An excellent tonic for the liver.
- ➤ Powerful blood purifier.
- ➤ Increases red blood cell count.
- ➤ Fights anaemia and detoxifies the body.
- ➤ Arrests the growth of harmful bacteria.
- ➤ Boosts the immune system.
- ➤ Increases energy levels almost instantly.
- ➤ Reduces varicose veins.
- ➤ Alkalinity helps neutralize acids and toxins.
- ➤ Washes drug deposits from the body.
- ➤ Rapid absorption and assimilation of nutrients into the body.
- ➤ Stimulates metabolism.

Because of its highly concentrated life force, start with as little as 25ml per day and slowly increase the intake, if desired. Although, wheat grass is available in bottled drinks and tablets, I suggest the approach of 'grow it and mow it'. The natural, fresh, home-grown wheatgrass juice is far superior in quality and far cheaper than commercial wheatgrass products.

How to grow and juice wheat grass

It couldn't be easier to grow wheat grass (and other grasses such as spelt and barley):

- ➤ Obtain a simple growing tray or pot and put about an inch or two thick of potting compost into it.
- ➤ Soak seeds for 12-24 hours.
- ➤ Sprinkle a liberal amount of seeds evenly across the soil.

- ➤ Cover lightly with more soil.

- ➤ Keep the soil moist (but do not make it sodden) and preferably keep the tray in a warm and sunny place.

- ➤ Cover the seeds and soil with some newspaper until the process of germination is complete and sprouts of grass appear.

- ➤ Harvest the grass when it reaches 6-8 inches tall (usually about 8 days).

- ➤ Let the grass grow for a second flush and harvest again (usually about 6 days).

- ➤ The root-bound soil can be broken up, mixed with compost and used again.

The traditional juicer costs from £35 and is suitable for small-scale juicing. The commercially marketed juicers are available from

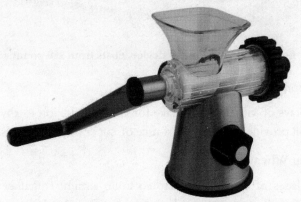

Fig. 5.16 A hand operated wheatgrass juicer

larger heath shops and start from £150. Alternatively, use a stone chutney grinder and strain the mulch through some cloth. Do not use electric blenders for juicing as the rapid blade movement causes

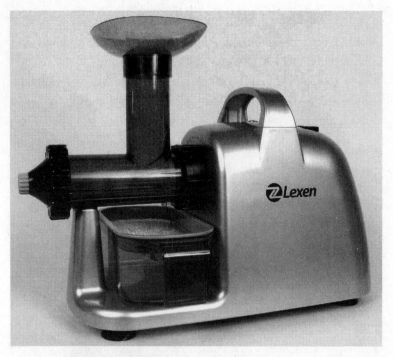

fig. 5.17 A home juicing device, costs from 150 pounds

oxidation of the chlorophyll.

Trays of vibrant grass make for a lovely addition to any house and will provide a very cheap source of super food goodness.

Storing Wheat grass juice

The blades of grass can be stored in an airtight container in the fridge for about three days, however the juice should be stored in a fridge and consumed within three hours. I have recently started to save my wheat grass juice as ice cubes and adding them to my juices when I feel like it; freezing the juice is said not to diminish its

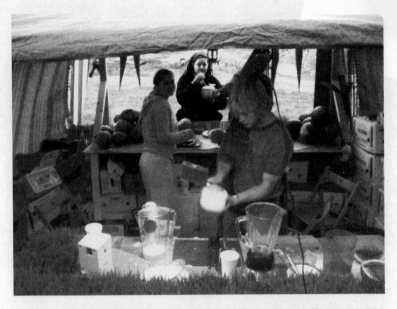

Fig. 5.18 Wheatgrass juice and coconut stall

potency too much and is very convenient for people who don't want to be growing it all the time.

My friends Pavla (pictured above on the left) and Dara ran a successful Wheat grass juice and Coconut stall at two festivals in the UK over the summer of 2006. When I asked Dara about his experiences at the festivals, he was enthusiastic in his reply:

'It was a real eye-opener - we completely sold out in two days. The people were so grateful that we were providing these lovely juices. It really hit home how good these simple drinks are, when we ran out of stock; people were pleading with us to get some more but it was not possible!'

Quick & healthy recipe ideas

The simplest snacks and meals are often the healthiest and tastiest. The recipes that follow are relatively quick and cheap to prepare.

HUMUS
(Serves 3+ people)

- ➤ 1 tin of chick peas (or some raw chick peas if you want to soak and boil them yourself)
- ➤ 1 large lemon (juicy)
- ➤ 1 large (or 2 small) garlic cloves (crushed).
- ➤ 150g of tahini
- ➤ 4-6 table spoons of hemp oil (or extra virgin olive oil)
- ➤ 2 pinches of sea/crystal salt
- ➤ A third of a level teaspoon of cayenne pepper
- ➤ A dash of cold water (to the consistency you like)

Blend all the ingredients until smooth, cover and store in the fridge. Humus is a wonderfully tasty, versatile and healthy food. Spread on toast and crackers, use as a dip for carrot or celery sticks, add to a salad-filled pitta or just nibble with a spoon. Altering the ratio of ingredients or adding new ones, such as avocado or spirulina can create many different varieties of humus.

VEGETABLE SALAD
(Serves 4-8 people)

> 3 tomatoes
> 2 large carrots
> One red onion
> 2 handfuls of sprouts
> Half an iceberg lettuce (washed)
> 1 small green pepper
> Juice of half an organic lemon
> 6 table spoons of hemp/extra virgin olive oil
> Pinch of ground rock/sea salt
> Pinch of cayenne pepper

Finely chop all the vegetables and mix together in a large bowl. Excellent accompaniment to a meal, as a sandwich filler or snack in it's own right. Other ingredients that go well in salads include seeds, beans, yoghurt, nuts, sliced apple and fresh herbs.

FRUIT SALAD WITH YOGHURT, NUTS AND HONEY
(Serves 2 people)

> 2 apples
> 2 bananas
> Natural set yoghurt
> Mixed nuts/seeds
> Honey

Finely slice the apples and bananas, mix and place in a bowl. Put the yoghurt on top, followed by some nuts or seeds and finally pour on the honey. If you are feeling very hungry, add museli or oats at the bottom of the bowl with a dash of goats milk. Other fruits, which go well in a fruit salad, include seedless grapes, papayas, mangoes and berries. Further ingredients could be soaked hemp seeds, spirulina powder or dried figs.

HEMP/OLIVE OIL/SPIRULINA ON TOAST

Drizzle hempseed oil on toast and sprinkle spirulina powder on top.

(Olive oil can be used instead of hempseed oil)

BROCCOLI DIPPED IN SALT/OLIVE OIL

Cut some broccoli into small florets and serve next to 2 small bowls; one with salt inside and the other with olive oil. Lightly dip the broccoli into the salt and then into the olive oil before eating raw.

HEMP-SPIRULINA SMOOTHIE
(Serves 3-5 people)
Ingredients:
- 3 organic bananas
- 3 tablespoons of hempseed oil (olive oil or coconut oil can be used if hempseed oil is not available)
- Half a cup of soaked hempseeds
- 2 tablespoons of apple cider vinegar
- 2 teaspoons of spirulina
- 8 soaked organic almonds
- 8 soaked organic dates
- Pinch of real salt
- Water (to desired consistency)

Blend and serve chilled.

Using a base of natural yoghurt and/or water and honey, it is easy to make smoothies that are very healthy and tasty. The cheap, hand held style of blenders are often the quickest to use and clean and start at around £10.

Adding hempseed oil will make them even healthier and tastier.

Popular fruits for smoothies are apples, bananas, strawberries, mangos, papaya, melon, grapefruit and pineapple.

The juice of fresh fruits can be mixed with water, honey, oils etc or simply drunk on their own. The vegetables can also be blended, with carrot juice being a favourite amongst juicing enthusiasts.

EMPEROR JUICE

(Serves 4-6 people)

This recipe takes a fair bit of preparation but the results are surely worth it; it is the most powerful and invigorating juice I've ever made!

- ➤ 1kg organic carrots
- ➤ 500g organic celery
- ➤ 1 organic lemon
- ➤ 1 chunk of organic ginger
- ➤ 1 tray of fresh wheat grass
- ➤ 1 tray of sprouted mung beans
- ➤ 2 tablespoons of spirulina
- ➤ 4 tablespoons of hempseed oil
- ➤ 2 tablespoons of apple cider vinegar
- ➤ Pinch of Himalayan crystal salt

> ➤ Pinch of organic cayenne pepper

Blend and serve cold

REJUVELAC

Rejuvelac is a mildly fermented wheat berry drink that is a highly important living food - drink. Rejuvelac can play a vital role in restoring health as it contains all the nutritional nourishment of

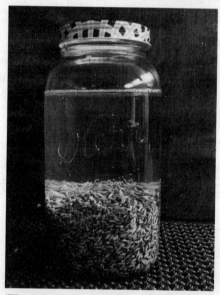

Fig. 5.19 Jar for Rejuvelac Preparation

wheat, yet is far more easily digested. It contains the bacteria that are necessary for a healthy colon and to remove toxins. It is also filled with vitamins B complex, C and E.

It was a food chemist named Harvey Lisle, who did the extensive research on Rejuvelac's contents and he found that Rejuvelac is rich in proteins, carbohydrates, dextrines, phosphates, saccharins, lactobacilli, and aspergillis oryzae. There are Amylases enzymes derived from aspergillis oryzae which have the faculty of breaking down large molecules of glucose, starch, and glycogens.

You can make Rejuvelac from any cereal grains, including barley, oats, rye, wheat, unshelled millet, brown rice (any whole grain rice), and raw unshelled buckwheat. For the best quality Rejuvelac, make sure to use fresh organically grown grains. Also keep everything clean. If using tap water, boil it for 3-5 minutes then let it cool before use. The Rejuvelac making container should be sterilized with boiling water.

How to make Rejuvelac

> Wash one cup of unpolished wheat thoroughly

> Soak in 5 cups of water

> Leave for 48 hours

> After 48 hours drain off the liquid into another container

> To this liquid add 2-3 teaspoons of honey

> Store in the refrigerator

> When serving add a squeeze of lemon juice

> Add 5 cups of water to the wheat remaining in the first container

> Repeat steps 4 to 7 (leave for only 24 hours this time)

> Add 5 cups of water to the wheat remaining in the first container

> Leave for 24 hours

> Drain the liquid into another container as before, adding honey. Store and serve as before

> The wheat remaining should now be discarded – or used as manure for the soil

NB: Diabetics can have small quantities but only in a diluted form.

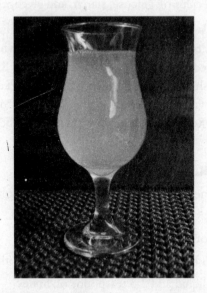

Fig. 5.20 A glass of delicious and nutritious Rejuvelac.

Light eating

Here in the West, most of us are eating far too much food each day and I've noticed many people in the East who are also over indulging.

Digestion is an extremely taxing process for the body to undergo, especially when cooked and denatured foods are being eaten regularly. Heavy digestion is the main reason why many of us need seven to nine hours of sleep each night and also a contributing factor to many afflictions such as lethargy, headaches and disease in general.

In western culture we have many myths concerning food. For example:

'Eat 3 square meals a day' implying that a balanced diet should consist of breakfast, lunch and dinner. Contrary to this belief, Indian yogic teachings state that a man who eats 3 times a day is indeed a `bhogi` or sick man. The man who eats twice a day is said to be a `rhogi` or `enjoyer of the senses` and the man who eats once a day is a `yogi`. Certainly, people who eat only one meal a day have high energy levels, are much healthier, live for longer and need less sleep.

"We need to eat food every day to be healthy", is another untruth of this age. The biological energy is carried within food but it is also carried within the rays of light and the air. It is entirely possible to dramatically cut food consumption without losing any energy, clarity of mind or health in general.

Dr. Jonathon Dao in his book 'The Ten Commandments of Health' mentions a study that involved interviewing two thousand people who were over one hundred years old. Concerning these people's eating habits, the researchers said:

'On reviewing nearly two thousand reported cases of persons who lived more than a century, we generally find some peculiarity of diet or habits to account for the alleged longevity; we find some were living amongst all the luxuries life could afford, others in the most abject poverty, begging their bread, some were samples of symmetry and physique while others were cripples, some drank large quantities of water, others little; some were total abstainers from alcoholic drinks, others drunkards; some smoked tobacco, others did not; some lived entirely on vegetables, others ate a great deal of animal foods; some lead active lives, others working more with their brains, others with their hands; some ate one meal per day, others four or five;...we notice great divergences in both habits and diet, but in those cases where we have been able to obtain a reliable account of the diet, we find one great cause which accounts for the majority of causes of longevity; moderation in the quantity of food!'

Other studies conducted in Europe during the Second World War showed that the general health of the population increased during times of food shortage. These studies indicate that in fact, we don't need as much food as we think we do in order to be healthy and that the body prefers a simple diet.

According to the Dr. Herbert Shelton and the Natural Hygiene movement, the total daily amount of food consumed should be the minimal amount, the appetite can be happy with (to avoid toxic accumulation and energy loss) for maximum longevity.

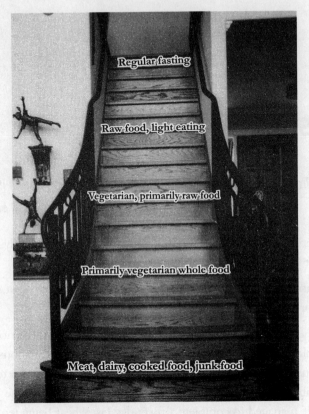

Fig. 5.21 The stairway to health

As the diagram above shows, attaining the highest health is not about taking new things into the body and spending lots of money. It is about incrementally ceasing to consume those things that the body does not require and was not designed to consume.

Fasting

'Prayer takes you to the door of the Lord; fasting opens it'

- Sufi saying

Perhaps the ultimate weapon against disease and catalyst for radiant health is the practice of fasting.

Fasting can be defined as: 'The act or practice of abstaining from or eating very little food.'

The practice of fasting seems to have been with us since the beginning of time. Ancient scriptures from various traditions and religions pay tribute to the power of fasting in no uncertain terms. The bible contains many references to fasting and of course Jesus himself managed to complete a forty-day fast whilst being tempted in the wilderness. According to Sathya Sai Baba, Jesus was also a very light eater, taking only one small meal per day.

Aside from its spiritual benefits, fasting is a key to physical health as it gives the body the rest and respite it needs to periodically purge itself of accumulated toxins. Our, natural doctors and healthcare professionals agree that in many cases, fasting is quick and highly effective way to facilitate healing; yet it takes discipline to undergo a fast and most people are not willing to give it a try. Good food is comforting and pleasant to eat yet the act of digestion and metabolism is extremely taxing for the body. Indeed, in the bible it is written:

> *'But food does not bring us near to God...'*
>
> *- I Corinthians 8:8a*

Philippus Paracelsus, the famous Swiss physician is considered one of three fathers of Western medicine, along with Greece's Hippocrates and Galen. Nearly 500 years ago, he expressed he's opinion of fasting:

> *'Fasting is the greatest remedy - the physician within!'*

It is the toxic debris and wastes of metabolism (from the biological process of converting food into living matter and the matter into energy) that bring about many of the physical ailments and premature aging. The food we eat needs to be:

➤ Masticated

➤ Digested

➤ Assimilated

➤ Eliminated

The four organs of elimination are:

➤ The bowels

➤ The kidneys

➤ The lungs

➤ The skin

In order for these organs to work perfectly, the body must

have high 'vital energy/chi/prana' levels, yet regularly eating food (especially cooked food) inevitably leads to a depletion of this energy. When vital energy drops below a certain point, this can be called 'enervation' and this is a main cause of ill health (physical as well as mental, emotional and spiritual).

I have personally enjoyed my experiences of fasting over the years and can vouchsafe that the vital energy levels do indeed get a powerful boost as a result. Some years ago I had a fasting experience that proved to me how effective it was simply to stop eating for a few days and instead just drink water. On the third day, I suddenly had to rush to the toilet to throw up. I made it just in time to grip on to the sides of the sink and projectile vomit what seemed to be gallons of a foul, acidic thick yellow liquid. I'm sure I nearly ripped the sink clean off the wall! After I had finished throwing-up, I brushed my teeth and sat down to meditate and calm down. My whole body erupted into a state of intense electrical tingling which felt very strange but not unpleasant; actually it felt very liberating. All the hairs on my body were standing up and it felt like surely a massive surge of released vital energy had been released. At that time I had been drinking about four cups of coffee per day and I knew after the experience that it was no doubt all that nasty toxic black caffeine that was coming out; if someone had have even said the word 'coffee' at that point I think I would have thrown-up again. A great burden had been lifted from my body.

There is a thirty-foot tube that connects the mouth to the rectum and it uses up a great deal of energy to pass food through its length. Readers will know that eating a large cooked meal can sometimes lead to an almost overwhelming tiredness. On the other hand, fasting can lead to a state of extremely high energy and well-being. By fasting we give our body a physiological rest and this rest builds up that vital energy. This newly liberated energy helps us to quickly expel our accumulated toxins. The body literally starts to clean itself, much in the same way as a housewife might start giving the house a thorough clean when the husband goes off for a few days with the kids. Why? Because it's a job she's wanted to do for a while but hasn't had the time or space to do it.

A test to see if you are in good health is to do a fast for two or three days. If you get headaches, nausea, foul smelling breath, dark urine or a white coating on the tongue, it means that your body is clogged up with decaying and un-eliminated toxic materials.

Every animal in the wilderness instinctively knows about fasting, in fact it is the only method they use to overcome illness. It seems that modern civilisation has caused us humans to lose our instinct to fast unless the situation is very serious, in which case our body will regurgitate whatever is attempted to be eaten.

I learned an important lesson a few years ago when I watched a two-year-old kid sitting in his highchair at breakfast time. His well-meaning parents were desperately trying to cajole the child into eating food when clearly he didn't want to. They would try to push the spoon in his mouth and he would turn his head away saying 'No!'. This drama went on until the child saw fit to throw the unwelcome food on the floor. If his body needed food at that early hour of the morning, he would happily eat. To me it was obvious that he shouldn't be forced to eat, however his parents became angry and began issuing threats such as 'if you don't eat your breakfast you won't be allowed to play today'…the story is an old one. Most of us were told to eat food regularly to 'keep our strength up', this has been our social conditioning and foolishly this poor advice gets passed down through generations and (more recently) backed-up by 'vested interest' research/lobby groups through the mass media and educational institutes.

SOME BENEFITS OF FASTING

> ➤ Increased energy and vitality
> ➤ Improved memory and cognitive processing
> ➤ Mental clarity
> ➤ Purging of bodily toxins
> ➤ Blood and lymph cleansing
> ➤ Increased elasticity of skin
> ➤ Brighter eyes
> ➤ Healthier, shiny hair
> ➤ Saves money (on food, washing up liquid, toilet paper etc)
> ➤ Increased chance of meaningful dreams, inspirations etc.
> ➤ Helps break addictions and bad habits
> ➤ Develops discipline
> ➤ Aids spiritual communion

According to Natural Hygiene advocate Dr Herbert Shelton, the body enters in the state of autolysis or self-digestion in about the fourth day of a fast in which the body can break down even cancerous tissues and eliminate them. In similar ways, many other serious illnesses can be overcome with fasting.

A fast can be partial or complete. 'A 'complete' fast is when no food at all is eaten.' It is a very potent way to cleanse the body. On the other hand a partial fast is easier and safer for the beginner.

It is the proven fact that when food intake is stopped or reduced, accumulated toxins begin to release, especially through the pores in the skin. The body is free to begin cleansing itself, as it no longer has to expend so much energy on digestion.

If you are new to fasting, you may initially experience some negative side effects, particularly if you are not generally a healthy eater. These side effects are usually mild and are a good sign that a purging of toxins is taking place. These side effects (and others) are the reason why many people do not succeed with fasting. The benefits far outweigh the early side effects which are listed so they can be anticipated and prepared for:

Physical: Itchy skin/scalp, headaches, nausia, fatigue, foul smelling breath, skin odour, dizziness, skin eruptions, white/yellow/grey coating on the tongue, strong smelling urine and stools, flatulence.

Emotional : irritability, insecurity etc.

Mental: Inability to concentrate or focus properly.

However, if urine is regularly drunk during the fast, the above healing responses are minimised or completely absent, thanks to the homeostasis promoting nature of urine.

TYPES OF FAST AND LIGHT EATING PRACTICES

Complete fast

During observing this, eat nothing at all and allow yourself only water or herbal tea to drink. This fast should be tried for only 24-48 hours if you are new to the practice as the detoxification can be very intense.

Urine fast

As above, with the addition of drinking some fresh urine each time you go to the toilet. This technique is highly recommended for many reasons (see the Urine Therapy chapter).

Grain fast

This system is popular in the yogic tradition. Organic oats simmered gently in pure water for 30 minutes and taken twice per day is a popular fast.

Fruit diet

The `fruitarian` diet can very quickly lead to increased energy and weight loss as well as a purging of bodily toxins. Eat only fruit (perhaps with some yoghurt and honey if desired).

One meal diet

Limit your intake of food to only one healthy meal, ideally in the early afternoon.

Raw food diet

Limit your intake to solely raw foods such as salads, fruit, sprouted grains and nuts.

The first meal after fasting should be light and healthy to avoid shocking the bodily system, so avoid gorging on heavy foods after you break fast. A vegetable juice or simple light salad is a beneficial way to break a fast.

Importantly, fasting is a key aspect of many religions, cultures and mystery teachings all over the world. From the Muslim Ramadan (which involves a month of partial fasting) to Jesus in the wilderness, the act of sacrificing the urge to eat in the name of God/salvation/evolution/purification is indeed a powerful tool that we can use any time we want. All we need is a little knowledge and some discipline. Rumi, the famous Sufi saint of the thirteenth century would impart eternal wisdom by way of poems which are now well documented and published all over the world. His opinion of fasting was clear.

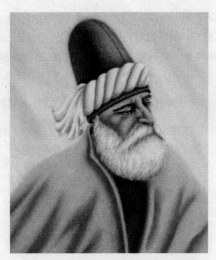

Fig. 5.22 Muslin Prophet (Rumi)

'There's hidden sweetness in the stomach's emptiness.

We are flutes, no more, no less.

If the soundbox is stuffed full of anything, no music.

If the brain and belly are burning clean with fasting, every moment a new song comes out of the fire.

The fog clears, and new energy makes you run up the steps in front of you.

Be emptier and cry like reed instruments cry.

Emptier, write secrets with the reed pen.

When you're full of food and drink, Satan sits where your spirit should, an ugly metal statue in place of the Kaaba.

When you fast, good habits gather like friends who want to help.

237

*Fasting is Solomon's ring. Don't give it to some illusion and lose
your power, but even if you have, if you've lost all will and control,
they come back when you fast, like soldiers appearing out of the
ground, pennants flying above them.*

A table descends to your tents, Jesus' table.

*Expect to see it, when you fast, this table spread with other food,
better than the broth of cabbages.'*

Testimonies

'I had spots on my face, was constantly blowing my nose, rarely had any energy and generally felt under the weather. James challenged me to follow his diet advice for one month and I accepted. Wow! What a change…I can't believe how quickly I felt better. My skin looks fine now and I have energy and enthusiasm about life. I like healthy eating now and will carry on for sure. Thanks.'

- Julian, London

'I had an annoying fungal infection that covered most of my toes and soles of my feet. James recommended that I drink a pint of hot water with salt, molasses and apple cider vinegar once or twice per day. He also recommended that I soak my feet in a bowl of hot water mixed with apple cider vinegar every day. It was nice to get some different advice from the usual creams and went out and bought the ingredients from the local supermarket. I followed the plan and the fungus issue was solved in about a week. Further more, my creaky joints in my knees and ankles stopped creaking too!'

- Jamal, Dorset

'I'd never thought about fasting before but after you mentioned it, I thought I'd try a three day complete fast. I only drank water and herbal tea for three days – and I'm so glad I stuck to it. I got many cravings, especially for toast and Marmite for some reason! – but by the evening of the second day I lost my desire to eat and instead felt amazingly relaxed and contented. I feel happier in my body now, lighter and more comfortable. I have lots more energy and at the moment no desire to eat any junk food again; my eyes are brighter and I feel stronger generally.'

- Daniel, London

'Learning how to fast was one of the best things I ever did. If ever I feel down, confused, toxified or sick, I simply do a one or two day fast and as if by magic I feel happier, healthier and more able to deal with whatever is going on in my life at the time. A little discipline is a small price to pay.'

- Jim, London

I followed the advice in the diet chapter of 'The Five Point Plan' by growing my own sprouts, taking super foods such as apple cider vinegar, hempseed oil and spirulina and noticed a huge difference in my energy levels (which was needed due to my high-stress job). I also noticed that apart from my physical health, I started to feel better in my self – both emotionally and mentally. I wouldn't give up my new diet for anything as it has changed my life considerably. Friends have also noticed that my skin has a glow to it and my eyes are brighter.

Tracy, London

Summary

Eat to live rather than live to eat. Know the difference between foods and drinks that are healthy and those that are unhealthy. Make your decisions based on a sound knowledge of nutrition and exercise discipline over any tendencies to consume too much or to consume poor quality products.

Eating a simple and limited diet of primarily raw foods is recommended for anyone seeking true health and well being.

EXERCISE

Regular exercise is an integral part of living a healthy, and happier life. This chapter contains some of the simplest and most effective exercises from the Indian, Chinese and Tibetan traditions.

Yoga Chi Kung

Over the last fifteen years I've developed my own system of internal and external exercise, which I call Yoga Chi Kung. It is generally a very calm and relaxing style of exercise that blends some of the safest, most gentle, most effective and most accessible aspects of the two art forms.

The following chart is an overview of the complete Level 1 syllabus.

Basics of yoga Preliminary notes 5 principles of yoga The benefits of yoga	Breathing exercises Circular breathing Cross breathing Sounding breath Bellows breathing	Yoga Philosophy Vedanta & Raja Yoga
Warm-ups Shoulder circling Knee circling Ankle circling	The Five Tibetan Rites Spinning Torso/leg raising	Great beings from India Sathya Sai Baba Shirdi Sai Baba

Neck stretching Hip circling/kidney massaging	Leaning back & forward Pushing up Cobra / dog	Babaji Meher Baba
Postures Salutation to the sun Triangle Inverse triangle Forward bend Dog Cat Locust Spine twist Cobblers Side stretch Hip stretch Hip strech 2 Child pose Death pose Plough Shoulder stand	Chi Kung Wu chi position Spine alignment Carrying the moon Zhan Zhuang Chi ball creation The Inner Smile	Meditation Basic meditation Light /Jyoti meditation
		Mudras Gyan Pran Apan Mritsanjeevini Linga

	Yogic diet	Yoga cleansing
	3 gunas Lacto vegetarianism Elixirs Fasting Urine therapy (Shivambu)	Neti
	Pranic healing Self healing	Mantra Sahana vavatu.. Om Gayatri Om Nama Shivaya Om Mane Padme Hum Sai Gayatri

Yoga

The word Yoga comes from the Sanskrit root 'Yog' which means 'to yoke' or 'to bind'. In this case, it refers to practice of binding man to God (atma to paramatma). It is the world famous and ancient practice of India that incorporates a wide variety of specialised physical, mental, emotional and spiritual practices.

Hatha Yoga refers to the physical aspects of yoga, namely postures (asana) and breathing exercises (pranamyama). Swami Sivananda (1854-1934) developed a classical Hatha Yoga system called Sivananda Yoga which is the best all round yoga system, I have come across and forms a basis for the Yoga Chi Kung system.

FIVE PRINCIPLES OF YOGA

The Five Principles of Yoga are the basis of attaining a healthy body and mind through the practice of Yoga.

Principle 1: Proper Relaxation

By releasing the tension in the muscles and putting the whole body at rest, you revitalize your nervous system (overcome 'enervation' and achieve inner peace. This relaxed feeling is carried over into all your activities and helps to conserve energy whilst letting go of all your worries and fears.

Principle 2: Proper Exercise

The physical body is designed to move and exercise. Proper exercise is achieved through the various postures of Yoga.

Principle 3: Proper breathing

This means breathing fully and rhythmically, making use of all the parts of your Lungs to increase your oxygen intake. Proper breathing should be deep, slow and rhythmical. Pranayama (breathing exercises) teaches how to recharge the body and control the mental state by regulating the flow of prana (life force).

Principle 4: Proper diet

A proper diet is one that nourishes both mind and body. It should be well balanced and based on natural foods. Proper diet in Yoga also means eating in moderation and eating only when you are hungry.

Principle 5: Positive thinking and meditation

Thoughts are to be controlled, if the yogi is to achieve success in yoga and life in general. Banishing damaging negative thoughts (such as angry responses or worrying) and controlling concentration/visualisation/detachment is achieved through the various meditation techniques.

Preliminary notes

STANDING

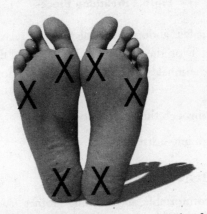

fig. 6.1 Weight balancing points on sole of feet

When standing upright on the feet, always remember to focus on balancing the body weight evenly between the three points. Avoid the temptation to tense the soles of the feet, as it will cause undue stress and instability in the posture.

Relax the feet and balance the weight.

BREATHING

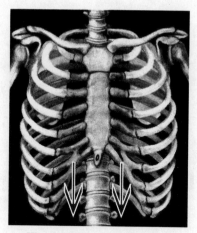

Fig. 6.2 Breathing Process

Take a 'firm-but-fair' abdominal inhalation and relax the diaphragm muscle completely on the exhalation. Do not hold the breath at the end of either the inhale or the exhale. This is known as 'circular' breathing.

Breathe gently through the nose if possible.

Exhale as you go into a stretch.

PREPARATION

> Wear comfortable, loose-fitting clothes (such as a T-shirt and tracksuit bottoms).

> Drink a small cup of water or herbal tea before practice.

> Make sure your body is clean.

> Go to the toilet before practice, if you can.

> Begin yoga practice with a short relaxation/meditation period.

EASY POSTURE

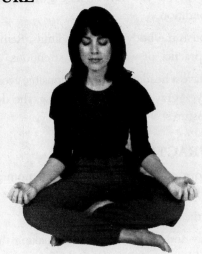

Fig. 6.3 Easy Posture

This Yoga Asana is one of the classic meditative poses. It helps to straighten the spine, slow down metabolism and still the mind. If you find that holding this pose is uncomfortable, place a folded blanket or cushion under the back of your buttocks. In order to stretch the leg muscles evenly, be sure to put each leg alternately on top. As you improve, move on to the half lotus and adept posture.

Keep your head and body straight. Relax the face muscles and shoulder muscles in particular. Breathe gently and close the eyes.

GENERAL CAUTIONS

> ➢ Do not practice any strenuous postures during the menstruation period.

> ➢ Do not drink any tea/coffee or eat any food before practice.

> ➢ Seek competent and professional medical advice regarding

251

yoga practice, if you have an illness of any sort, especially a heart condition.

> Never push the body beyond its limits. Remember that the correct practice of yoga is never strenuous.

> If you have a headache, cold or sinusitis, avoid any postures that may aggravate the condition e.g. the dog or shoulder stand postures.

AN ASANA PRACTICE SHOULD

> Reflect our condition at the present moment (know your own body).

> Fit into the time you have available.

> Be steady and comfortable while making the body strong and flexible.

> Emphasize the spine.

> Adapt to achieve your goal according to your individual capacity and limits.

> Proceed in intelligent orderly steps.

> Use the breath to adapt postures and integrate the body and mind.

Warm up exercises

SHOULDER CIRCLING

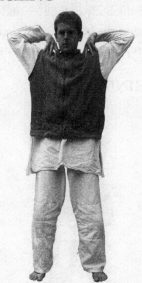

Fig. 6.4 Shoulder Circling

Place your fingers on your shoulders and point your elbows out at 90 degrees to the body. Draw large, slow circles with the elbows, as large as you can make them. Breathe in deeply on the way up and exhale fully on the way down. Resist the tendency to speed up the circles, slower is better.

Repeat 3-10 times in both directions.

KNEE CIRCLING

Place the feet together and hold on to your kneecaps with the palms of your hands. Slowly circle the knees whilst maintaining a firm grip with the hands. After a few repetitions, circle the knees the other way.

ANKLE CIRCLING

Balance the weight of the body on one leg and raise the knee of the other leg at 90 degrees to the body. Slowly circle the foot as wide as possible. After a few repetitions, repeat with the other foot.

NECK STRETCHING

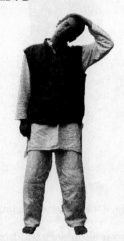

Fig. 6.5 Neck Stretching

Very gently hold on to the side of the head and exhale as you pull it down to the side. Breathe deeply and hold the position for at least thirty seconds. Repeat to the other side.

HIP CIRCLING / KIDNEY MASSAGE

Stand with the legs slightly apart and rub the palms of the hands together rigorously until they feel hot. Take a firm hold around the middle of the back (around the same area that the kidneys are situated) and circle the hips slowly in wide circles. Repeat a few times and reverse the direction.

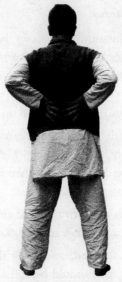

Fig. 6.6 Hip Circling

SALUTATION TO THE SUN

In Hindu mythology, the sun god is worshipped as a symbol of health and immortal life. The Rig Veda declares that 'Surya is the Soul, both of the moving and unmoving beings'. The Sun Salutation originated as a series of prostrations to the sun. Traditionally, it is performed at dawn, facing the rising sun. In time, each of the twelve positions came to have its own mantra, celebrating aspects of the sun's divinity. I feel that if only one aspect of Yoga is to be practiced, this is the one as it leads to all-over strength and flexibility marvellously.

The Sun Salutation is a graceful sequence of twelve positions performed as one continuous exercise. Each position counteracts the one before, stretching the body in a different way and alternately expanding and contracting the chest to regulate the breathing. On practicing daily, it will bring great flexibility to the spine and joints and lead to strong body. It is a great limbering-up exercise in preparation for the postures.

One round of Sun Salutation consists of two sequences, the first leading with the right foot in positions 4 and 9, the second leading with the left. Keep your hands in one place from positions 3 to 10 and try to co-ordinate your movements with your breathing. Start by practicing two rounds and gradually build up to twelve rounds.

> ➢ Stand erect with feet together and hands in the prayer position in front of your chest. Make sure your weight is evenly distributed. Exhale and bend forward slightly from the hips, keeping the back straight.

> ➢ Inhaling, stretch your arms up and arch back from the waist, pushing the hips out, legs straight. Relax your neck.

> ➢ Exhaling, fold forward, and hang down keeping the legs straight. Ideally, you should be able to touch your feet with your palms and touch the knees with your forehead.

> ➢ Inhaling, bring the left (or right) leg back and place the knee on the floor. Arch back and look up, lifting your chin.

> ➢ Retaining the breath, bring the other leg back and support your weight on hands and toes.

- Exhaling, lower your knees, then your chest and then your forehead, keeping your hips up and your toes curled under.

- Inhaling, lower your hips, point your toes and bend back. Keep legs together and shoulders down. Look up and back.

- Exhaling, curl your toes under; raise your hips and pivot into the 'dog' position. Try to push your heels and head down and keep your shoulders back.

- Inhaling, step forward and place the left (or right) foot between your hands. Rest the other knee on the floor and look up, as in position 4.

- Exhaling, bring the other leg forward and bend down from the waist, keeping your palms as in position 3.

- Inhaling, stretch your arms forward, then up and back over your head and bend back slowly from the waist, as in position 1.

- Exhaling, gently come back to an upright position and bring your arms down by your sides.

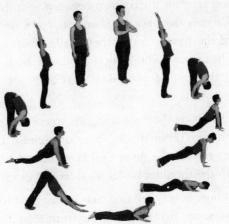

Fig. 6.7 Sun Salutation

Postures (asana)

CHILD POSTURE

Procedure

Kneel on the floor. Touch your big toes together and sit on your heels.

Exhale and lay your torso down between your thighs. Broaden your sacrum across the back of your pelvis and narrow your hip points toward the navel, so that they nestle down onto the inner thighs. Lengthen your tailbone away from the back of the pelvis while you lift the base of your skull away from the back of your neck.

Lay your hands on the floor alongside your torso, palms upward and fingers in the 'Gyan mudra' position; release the fronts of your shoulders toward the floor. Feel how the weight of the front shoulders pulls the shoulder blades wide across your back.

The child pose is very relaxing. Stay in this pose for at least one minute. To come up, first lengthen the front torso, and then with an inhalation lift from the tailbone as it presses down and into the pelvis.

Benefits

> ➢ Gently stretches the hips, thighs, and ankles.

> ➢ Calms the brain and helps relieve stress and fatigue.

> ➢ Relieves back and neck pain.

Cautions

Avoid this posture if you are suffering from Diarrhoea or knee injuries or in case you are pregnant.

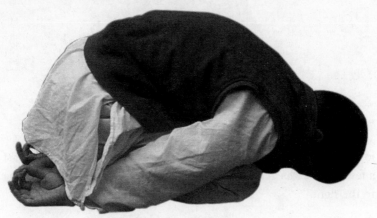

Fig. 6.8 Child Posture

TRIANGLE POSTURE

Procedure

Stand with your feet well apart. Point your left foot to the left, and your right foot at 90 degrees to your body. Stretch your arm out at shoulder level and bring the right arm straight up, against your right ear. Now inhale.

As you exhale, bend to the left and slightly forward to bypass your ribs. Slide your left hand down your left leg and hold on to the

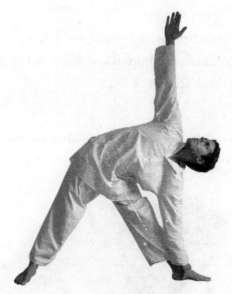

Fig. 6.9 Triangle Posture

lowest part you can reach. Look up at your right hand. Take at least a few full breaths in this position before releasing it. Repeat, bending to the right.

Benefits

- ➢ Stimulates blood flow.
- ➢ Helps to stretch and relax the back, shoulders, legs and arms.
- ➢ Increases the flow of blood to the head.
- ➢ Stretches the muscles of the thighs, calves and the hamstrings.
- ➢ The slight twist of the spine creates suppleness in the spinal discs and relieves lower back discomforts.

INVERSE TRIANGLE POSTURE

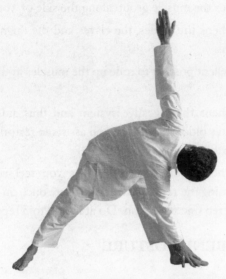

Fig. 6.10 Inverse Triangle Posture

Procedure

Stand with the feet together and the arms by your sides, inhale and spread your legs apart, slightly further than shoulder distance. Stretch your arms straight out from the shoulders parallel to the floor with your palms facing down. Exhale slowly and turn your right foot toward the right 90 degrees.

Place the palm of your left hand flat on the floor next to the outside of your right foot. Rest the right elbow on the outside of the right knee.

Stretch the right arm over your head, parallel with the floor, with the inside of the elbow resting on the ear. Hold for at least thirty seconds whilst breathing gently through the nostrils. Slowly return to a standing position and repeat on the other side.

Benefits

> ➤ Stretches the muscle group along the side of your torso.

> ➤ Strengthens the ankles, the claves and the thighs as well as the arms.

> ➤ An excellent posture to tone up the muscles in the waist and hips.

> ➤ Strengthens the digestive system and thus aids digestion, stimulates blood circulation and assists in restoring strength and flexibility to the spine.

> ➤ Hold the posture for as long as you feel comfortable. Performing the reverse triangle posture once on each side is considered one repetition. Do at least 1 to 3 repetitions.

FORWARD BEND POSTURE

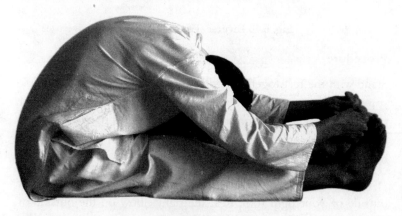

Fig. 6.11 Forward Bend Posture

Procedure

Sit on the floor with the legs together and extended straight out in front. Keep the back straight, shoulders level and head straight. Place the hands, palm down, flat on top of the thighs then inhale deeply. Exhale and extend the arms straight out in front, parallel with the floor with fingers pointed straight ahead and palms facing down.

Inhale slowly while raising the arms over the head, keeping them straight, and bending as far back as you feel comfortable. Tilt the head back and look up at the hands. Exhale slowly bending forward at the waist and grasp the feet with the hands. Bring the head as close to the knees as possible, placing it on the knees if you can, keeping the legs straight. (If you are unable to grasp the feet then grasp the ankles). Hold this position for the duration of the exhalation (hold for a few breaths if possible). Inhale slowly and return to the seated position.

Repeat this posture for two or three times holding each repetition for at least the duration of the exhaling breath and take a few deep breaths in-between each repetition. As you become more adept at doing the forward bend, you may begin breathing slowly through the nostrils while holding the posture to increase its duration.

Benefits

> All the vertebrae of the spine and each muscle in the back is stretched.

> The compression or contraction of the stomach followed by the release increases blood flow to the abdominal region and tones the muscles.

> Gas is released and sluggish digestion happens.

> Constipation gets improved.

> Stretches the muscles in the calves and thighs helping to relieve fatigue and soreness in the lower extremities.

DOG POSTURE

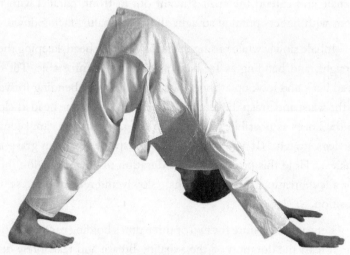

Fig. 6.12 Dog Posture

Procedure

Come onto the floor on your hands and knees. Set your knees directly below your hips and your hands slightly forward of your shoulders. Spread your palms, index fingers parallel or slightly turned out, and turn your toes under.

Exhale and lift your knees away from the floor. At first keep the knees slightly bent and the heels lifted away from the floor. Lengthen your tailbone away from the back of your pelvis and press it lightly toward the pubis. Against this resistance, lift the sitting bones toward the ceiling, and from your inner ankles draw the inner legs up into the groin.

Then, with an exhalation, push your top thighs back and stretch your heels onto or down towards the floor. Straighten your knees but be sure not to lock them. Firm the outer thighs and roll the upper thighs inward slightly. Narrow the front of the pelvis.

Tense the outer arms and press the bases of the index fingers firmly into the floor. From these two points lift along your inner arms from the wrists to the tops of the shoulders. Push your shoulder blades against your back, then widen them and draw them toward the tailbone. Keep the head between the upper arms; don't let it hang. Hold the position for at least ten breaths.

To finish, bend your knees to the floor with an exhalation and rest in the Child's pose for a while.

Benefits

> Calms the brain and helps relieve stress and mild depression.

> Energizes the body.

> Stretches the shoulders, hamstrings, calves, arches, and hands.

> Strengthens the arms and the legs.

> Helps relieve the symptoms of menopause.

> Relieves menstrual discomfort when done with the support of the head.

> Helps prevent osteoporosis.

> Improves digestion.

> Relieves headache, insomnia, back pain, and fatigue.

> Therapeutic for high blood pressure, asthma, flat feet, sciatica, sinusitis.

Cautions

Avoid this posture if you suffer from carpal tunnel syndrome, diarrhoea or are in late term pregnancy. If you have high blood pressure or a headache, support your head on a bolster or block, ears level between the arms.

CAT POSTURE

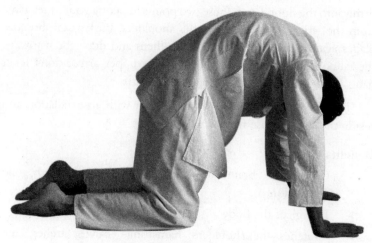

Fig. 6.13 (a) Cat Posture

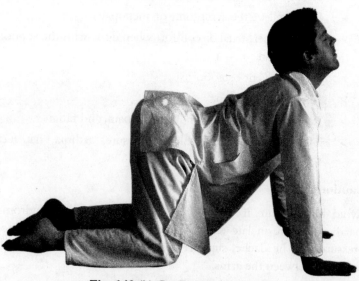

Fig. 6.13 (b) Cat Posture (curved)

This pose teaches to initiate movement from the centre and to coordinate movement and breath. These are two of the most important themes in asana practice. The alignment of your centre depends on the positioning of your pelvis. Therefore, think of your hip positioning as the centre of each pose.

Procedure

When you are ready to begin, breathe in deeply. As you exhale, turn your hips forward as in the first picture. Do this by gently pulling the abdominal muscles backward toward the spine, tucking the tailbone (coccyx) down and under, and gently contracting the buttocks. Press firmly downward with your hands in order to stay lifted out, of the shoulders; and press the middle of your back toward the ceiling, rounding your spine upward. Curl your head inward.

As you inhale, turn your hips the other way. Do this by releasing the grip of the buttocks, reversing the tilt of your pelvis, and curving your spine into a smoothly arched backbend. The pubic bone will move backward through the legs, the sitting bones will turn upward, and the sacrum will change its angle.

Keep the navel backward towards the spine as you do this, and continue pressing downward into your hands to lengthen the arms and stay lifted out of the shoulders. Lift your chest away from the waist, lift your head, slide the shoulder blades down your back, and either gaze at a point on the floor in front of you or upward towards the ceiling - or close your eyes and focus on the way your body feels.

Feel the flow of the curve. Increase the curve by tilting your pelvis more and moving the spine deeper into your back, bringing the curve up your back. Do this without sagging into the shoulders. Arch the full length of your spine to its maximum.

Benefits

- ➤ Loosens the back and the spine.
- ➤ Stretches the front and back of the body.
- ➤ Frees your neck and shoulders.
- ➤ Elongates your back muscles.
- ➤ Stimulates spinal fluid and the digestive tract.
- ➤ Improves circulation through the spine and core.
- ➤ Reduces stress.

SPINE TWIST POSTURE

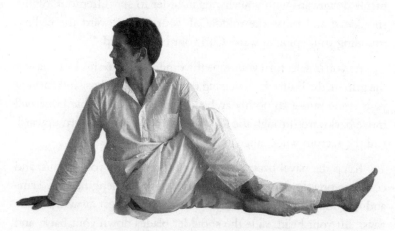

Fig. 6.14 (a) Spine Twist Posture on the ground

Procedure

Sit on the floor, with both legs out, keeping straight and back at 90 degrees to the floor. Bend the left, leg so the sole of the foot lies next to the right kneecap. Place the palm of the left hand on the floor behind you and exhale as you twist and look at the wall behind you. Hold for at least thirty seconds. Repeat the other side.

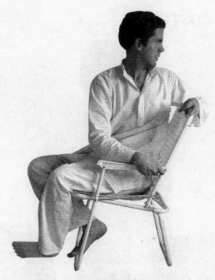

Fig. 6.14 (b) Spine Twist Posture on the chair

A simple alternative is to take a deep inhalation, hold on to the opposite kneecap with one hand, whilst gripping on to the chair. Exhale as you twist the spine and look behind you. This exercise is useful for people who have to spend a long time in the posture of sitting down in an office.

Benefits

> Loosens the spine from the coccyx to the base of the skull.

> Loosens the hips.

> Removes adhesions in the joints (rheumatism).

> Increases the synovial fluid of the joints.

> Tones the roots of the spinal nerves and the sympathetic nervous system.

> Massages abdominal muscles.

> Stimulates the gall bladder, spleen, kidneys, liver and bowels.

COBBLER'S POSTURE

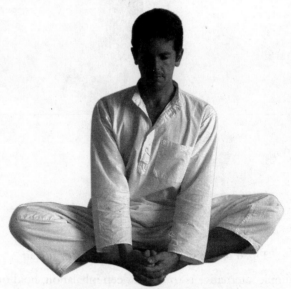

Fig. 6.15 (a) Cobbler's Posture

This asana is called the Cobbler's pose after the typical sitting position of Indian cobblers. It is an excellent groin and hip opener. In our Western culture, many people have tight hips from sitting in chairs and also from activities such as running, hiking, and biking. This pose is also an excellent preparation for childbirth and suggested during menstruation. Men and women can both benefit from the hip opening qualities of this asana postures. The kids often find it fun and easy to perform.

Procedure

Start with bare feet, sit with knees spread to the side and the soles of the feet together. Tighten the buttock muscles, pulling each one back and out to assure that sure you are sitting with equal weight on each of your sitting bones. With the pelvis positioned perpendicularly to

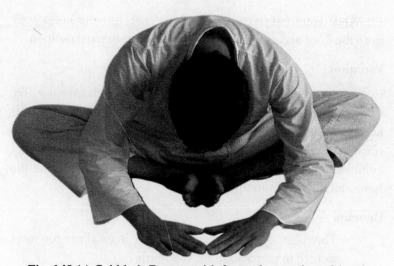

Fig. 6.15 (a) Cobbler's Posture with forward extension of head

the floor extend the spine as if a string were pulling you up to the sky from the top of your head.

As you sit with feet together grasp the feet with the hands and pull the heels as close toward the perineum as possible. Knees should aim toward the floor, letting the force of gravity slowly work its magic. The spine should extend up out of the pelvis with maximizing the space between the vertebrae and maintaining the 'normal' curves.

Those that have tight hamstring muscles may have difficulty in achieving a normal concave curve in their lumbar spine in their lower back. This is helped by sitting on one or more folded blankets with the sitting bones quite close to the front edge so that the pelvis is given a slight forward tilt.

Hold on to the feet. The upper thighs should roll to the outside as the femur extends out of the pelvis and the knees arc down to or towards the floor.

271

When you want to come out of the pose, lift your knees away from the floor and extend the legs back to their original position.

Variation

Extend the crown of the head forward with an extended spine. Try to keep normal spinal curves in your back. Imagine bringing your navel in front of your feet. Use bolsters or stacked fists to lean on if you do not reach the floor and want to. Remember to come forward by tilting the pelvis moving from the hip joints, not rounding the spine and moving from the waist.

Benefits

> This pose opens the hip joints. It is excellent for most women in preparation for childbirth.

> Creates stretch in the inner thighs, groins, and knees.

> Opening and freedom of the hips and thigh muscles.

> Chest opening and shoulders rolling back restores posture from sitting, computer use, and driving.

> Stimulates abdominal organs.

> Increases body circulation.

> May help relieve mild depression, anxiety, and fatigue.

> Soothing menstrual discomfort.

> May be useful for symptoms of menopause.

> Consistent practice of this pose until late into pregnancy is said to ease childbirth.

> Lifts energy and immune booster.

Cautions

This pose is usually contraindicated for women who have recently given birth.

Groin or knee injury: Place folded blankets or bolsters under your knees for support. Listen carefully to your body and stop if it hurts in a way that is burning.

SEATED SIDE STRETCH POSTURE

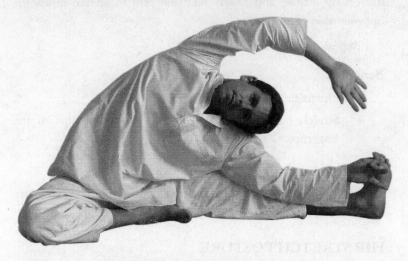

Fig. 6.16 Seated Side Stretch Posture

Procedure

From a seated position extend the right leg out 45 degrees towards the corner of the room. Bring the left foot in close proximity to the hips. Extend the right arm over the right leg with the right palm facing up.

Inhale and reach out for the left fingers up towards the ceiling, lifting out of the hips.

Exhale and arch over to the right, reaching out for the left fingers towards the right foot, bringing the left arm directly over the left ear.

Keep the left shoulder pressing back, allowing the chest to stay open and facing forward. Keep the chin off the chest, looking forward or up at the ceiling. Breathe and hold for a couple of seconds.

To release: Inhale and reach out for the left fingers up towards the ceiling, exhale and slowly take the arm in an arc down the opposite side of the body.

Repeat on other side.

Benefits

> Opens the hips.

> Stretches the side of the body - from the hips to the fingertips.

Caution

Do not practice this posture in the case of recent or chronic injury to the knees, hips, arms or shoulders.

HIP STRETCH POSTURE

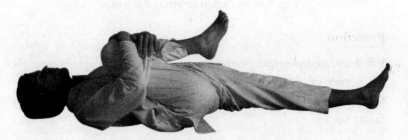

Fig. 6.17 (a) Hip Stretch Posture

Procedure

Lie down on your back and gently pull one knee towards the chest. Breathe deeply into the hips and groin area and hold for as long as you feel like. When finished, slowly lower the leg to the floor and repeat the same with the opposite leg.

This is a very relaxing pose which I particularly like to do before sleeping.

Benefits

> Relieves tension in the hips, groin and lower back area.

> Stretches the thigh muscles.

> Loosens the knees.

HIP STRETCH POSTURE 2

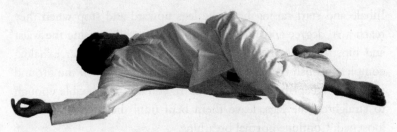

Fig. 6.17 (B) Hip Stretch Posture 2

Procedure

Lie on your back, bend the left knee and lay the left leg on the floor. Bring the right ankle of the left knee and place the right foot on the floor. Breathe deeply into the spine, hips and groin area. Hold for at least 30 seconds and repeat on the other side.

PLOUGH POSTURE

The Plough pose is my favourite. Although many people find it quite difficult at first, it is well worth the effort to practice it each day upon waking up in the morning and before bed.

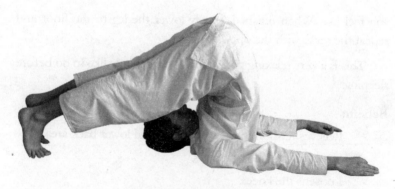

Fig. 6.18 Plough Posture

Procedure

Inhale and start raising both the legs upward and stop when they reach a 90 degree angle to the floor. Exhale whilst raising the waist and hips; pushing the legs up and over the head. After exhaling completely, push the legs further back and try to touch the ground with toes. Keep the toes stretched. If you are not flexible enough to straighten the legs, leave them bent until the hamstrings have loosened. Continue normal breathing.

In this position the head, the shoulders, the toes and the arms should rest on the ground. The chin pressed into the top of the chest and the tip of the tongue is pressed against the roof of the mouth.

Inhale and lift the toes of the floor keeping the legs straight. Continue inhaling and slowly lower the back to the ground, one vertebra after the other. Exhale and gently bring the legs back to the normal position.

This asana is difficult initially, especially for women with heavy hips and men with big tummies. This asana should be maintained for at least thirty seconds.

Benefits

> The spine is stretched fully in a curve. It becomes more elastic and its overall functioning is improved.

> All the muscles from toes to waist are also stretched, helping improvement in the functioning of veins. This asana is also useful for gastric troubles, and digestion problems.

> Helps to both wake up in the morning and get to sleep at night.

> Leads to a tremendous release of biological energy (prana) from the base of the spine.

Cautions

Avoid jerks or speedy movements as it might cause some injury to the backbone. The movements should be controlled at every stage of this asana.

People suffering from spleen and liver complaints should seek professional advice before practicing this asana.

SHOULDER STAND POSTURE

Procedure

Lie flat on your back. Inhale deeply while raising your legs and spine until the toes point to the ceiling. The body rests on the shoulders and the back of the neck. The body is supported by the hands, which are placed on the centre of the spine between the waist and the shoulder blades. Keep your spine and legs straight.

Breathe slowly and deeply with the abdomen and concentrate on the thyroid gland. On a male, the thyroid gland is located behind the Adams apple. For women, it is located in the same area which is a few inches above the sternal notch (hollow of the neck where the

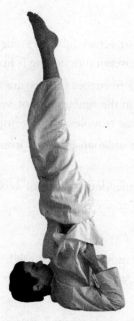

Fig. 6.19 Shoulder Stand Posture

neck joins the rest of the body.), or approximately half way up the neck from the sternal notch. Hold for 20 seconds to 2 minutes.

To come out of this posture, just bend your knees, curve your back and slowly return to lying on the floor while exhaling. First bend your knees, put the palms on the floor, then curving the spine, gradually unfold it the way one unrolls a carpet. When your entire back touches the floor, straighten the knees, take a deep breath and slowly lower your legs to the ground while breathing out.

Benefits

> Stimulates the thyroid gland to work at peak efficiency (the thyroid gland which is mainly responsible for your correct weight and youthful appearance).

- ➤ Regulates the sex glands.
- ➤ Vitalizes the nerves.
- ➤ Purifies the blood.
- ➤ Promote good circulation.
- ➤ Strengthens the lower organs and helps them to stay in place.
- ➤ Stretch to the neck muscles.
- ➤ Eases constipation, indigestion and asthma.
- ➤ Increases virility.
- ➤ Recommended for women after childbirth and for those suffering from painful menstruation and other disorders.

Caution

Do not practice this if you are suffering from organic disorders of the thyroid gland. Be very cautious if you are suffering from chronic nasal catarrh.

Check list of things to remember when holding a yoga posture:

- ➤ Am I breathing correctly?
- ➤ Are my limbs relaxed and in the correct position?
- ➤ Is my body in the correct position?
- ➤ Am I tensing any muscles unnecessarily?
- ➤ Is my mind calm?

Breathing exercises (Pranayama)

Breathing is so simple and so obvious we often take it for granted; ignoring the power it has to affect body, mind and spirit. With each inhale we bring oxygen into the body and spark the transformation of nutrients into fuel. During exhalation we purge the body of carbon dioxide, a toxic waste. Breathing also affects our state of mind. It can make us excited or calm, tense or relaxed. It can make our thinking confused or clear. Also, in the yogic tradition, air is the primary source of prana or life force, a psycho-physio-spiritual force that permeates all of creation.

Pranayama is loosely translated as prana/breath control. The ancient yogis developed many breathing techniques to maximize the benefits of prana. Pranayama is used in yoga as a separate practice to help clear and cleanse the body and mind. It is also used in preparation for meditation and during the postures to maximise the benefits.

SOUNDING BREATH

The sounding breath is sometimes called the 'Darth Vader' breath. It involves constricting the back of the throat while breathing to create an 'ah' sound.

Procedure

Come into a comfortable seated position with your spine erect, or lie down on your back. Begin taking long, slow, and deep breaths through the nostrils.

Allow the breath to be gentle and relaxed as you slightly contract the back of your throat, creating a steady hissing sound as you breathe in and out. The sound need not be forced, but it should be loud enough so that if someone came close to you they would hear it.

Lengthen the inhalation and the exhalation as much as possible without creating tension anywhere in your body, and allow the sound of the breath to be continuous and smooth.

To help create the proper 'ah' sound, hold your hand up to your mouth and exhale as if trying to fog a mirror. Inhale in the same way. Notice how you constrict the back of the throat to create the fog effect. Now close your mouth and do the same thing while breathing through the nose.

Benefits

> ➢ Focuses the mind
> ➢ Increases mindfulness
> ➢ Generates internal heat

COMPLETE BREATHING

The 'complete' or 'three-part' breath teaches us how to fill the three chambers of the lungs, beginning with the lower lungs, then moving up through the thoracic region and into the clavicular region.

Procedure

Sit with your spine erect, or lay down on your back. Begin by taking long, slow, and deep breaths through the nostrils. As you inhale, allow the belly to fill with air, drawing air deep into the lower lungs. As you exhale, allow the belly to deflate like a balloon. Repeat several times, keeping the breath smooth and relaxed, and never straining. Repeat several times.

Breathe into your belly and also expand the mid-chest region by allowing the rib cage to open outward to the sides. Exhale and repeat several times.

Follow the first two steps and continue inhaling by opening the upper chest. Exhale and repeat. Combine all three steps into one continuous or complete flow.

Benefits

> ➤ Promotes proper diaphragmatic breathing.
> ➤ Relaxes the mind and the body.
> ➤ Oxygenates the blood and purges the lungs of residual carbon dioxide.

CROSS BREATHING

Cross breathing (nadi shodhana – 'the sweet breath') is the simple form of alternate nostril breathing, suitable for beginners and advanced students. 'Nadi' means channel and it refers to the energy pathways through which prana flows. 'shodhana' means cleansing and nadi shodhana means channel cleaning.

Procedure

Hold your right hand up and curl your index and middle fingers toward your palm.

Place your thumb next to your right nostril and your ring finger and little finger by your left.

Close the left nostril by pressing gently against it with your ring finger and little finger and inhale through the right nostril. The breath should be slow, steady and full.

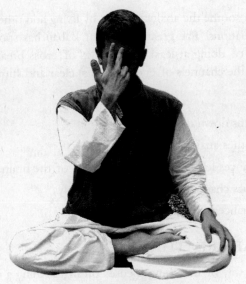

Fig. 6.20 Cross Breathing

Now, close the right nostril by pressing gently against it with your thumb, and open your left nostril by relaxing your ring finger and little finger exhaling fully with a slow and steady breath.

Inhale through the left nostril, close it, and then exhale through the right nostril.

That's one complete round of nadi shodhana.

> Inhale through the right nostril.
> Exhale through the left.
> Inhale through the left.
> Exhale through the right.

Begin with five to ten rounds and add more as you feel ready. Remember to keep your breathing slow, easy and full.

Nadi shodhana helps you control your stress and anxiety. If you start to feel stressed out, ten or so rounds will help calm you down.

It also helps soothe the anxiety caused by flying and other fearful or stressful situations. The great Mahavatar Babaji has spoken of the importance of doing at least three cycles of cross breathing every day to keep the channels of energy (nadis) clear and stimulated.

Benefits

> Calms down the mind.

> Soothes anxiety and stress.

> Balances left and right hemispheres of the brain.

> Clears channels of energy in the body.

> Enhances clear thinking.

CIRCULAR BREATHING

This simple way of breathing focuses on maintaining a connection between inhale and exhale whilst making sure not to hold the breath in between.

Take a 'firm but fair' inhalation and completely relax the diaphragm muscle (at the top of the abdominal area) during the exhalation.

Benefits

> The body gets filled with energy and is nourished as it receives more oxygen than it is accustomed to.

> Toxins are released from the muscles and cells, and exhaled.

> As the body and cells are cleansed and energized, they also release emotional and mental 'toxins' that are the result of emotions and traumas that have been suppressed and held in the body.

Learning to breathe in a gentle, circular way takes disciplined and much self-reminding measures however the benefits are well worth the effort.

BELLOWS BREATHING

Bellows breathing consists primarily in forced rapid breaths. Although air is forced both in and out, emphasis is placed on the expulsion or explosion of air. A series of such expulsions, each following the other in quick succession without pause, either full or empty, may be called 'a round.' One expulsion (followed by a quick inhalation) should last for only half a second or less. Beginners should keep a round to about five expulsions although the number may be increased to ten, or to any number needed to obtain the desired effect.

Benefits

> Increased ventilation.
>
> Increased blood circulation.
>
> Increased clearing of nasal passages.
>
> Increased thinking capacity.
>
> Pacification of mental disturbances.

Try to limit breathing to the nostrils only. After a few rounds of bellows breathing, take a deep breath in and then relax for a few moments.

This breathing exercise is best done in a seated position, allowing maximum relaxation of abdominal muscles and easy diaphragmatic breathing.

Caution

Excessive ventilation through yoga breathing exercises results in light heartedness, giddiness or a feeling of floating in the air. Always stay within your comfort limits and never push too hard.

Meditation (Dhyana)

Meditation is a focusing of the mind on a single object, thought or sound which eventually leads to the ending of all thought. As thoughts dissipate, the mind becomes quiet, and we are able to be fully in the present moment - or the 'eternal now'. The techniques of meditation are simple and easy to learn, but the ability to keep the mind focused takes time, patience and practice. The benefits of a regular meditation practice include reduction of stress, tension, anxiety and frustration, as well as improved memory, concentration, inner peace and well being of our entire body.

TECHNIQUE FOR YOGA MEDITATION

At first sit in a comfortable position, either cross-legged on the floor or in a chair. Be carefull you sit up tall with the spine straight, the shoulders relaxed and the chest open. Then rest the hands on the knees with the palms facing up. Lightly touch the index finger to the thumb. Relax the face, jaw, and belly. Let the tongue rest on the roof of the mouth, just behind the front teeth. Allow the eyes to retain lightly close.

Breathe slowly, smoothly and deeply in and out through the

nose. Let the inhale start in the belly and then rise gently up into the chest. As the breath slows and deepens, let go of any thoughts or distractions and allow the mind to focus on the breath. Feel the breath as it moves in and out of the body, feeling it move through the nose, throat, windpipe and lungs. Feel the body as it rises and falls with each breath. Bring as much of your awareness and attention to your body and breath as possible with each moment. As the thoughts return to the mind, observe them and then let them go, and return the focus back to the body and breath.

Practice this meditation for 5-20 minutes. To end, gently let the eyes blink open, inhale and rub the palms together in front of the heart, exhale and gently bow. Take a moment or two before moving on with the rest of your day.

It is written in the 'Hatha Yoga Pradipika': "The Yogi, who seated in Padmasana (cross legged posture), inhales through the entrances of the nadis (biological channels of energy) and fills them with vital air gains liberation". This might sound a bit esoteric to many readers, but I, yoga practitioners and meditators around the world seem to agree that indeed there are benefits to regular practice, which could definitely lead to some kind of 'liberation' - perhaps liberation from negative or distorted thoughts, perhaps liberation from stress and tension and perhaps even liberation from the wheel of rebirth known as 'samsara'.

If you don't fancy sitting upright to meditate, you can practice it lying down before you fall asleep at night or before your siesta. The trick is to simply observe the thoughts going through your head (and then let them go) and focus on your breathing. This is called 'conscious breathing' - being aware at all times that you are breathing. Seems like a simple thing to do however the results can be quite amazing. You may find that this practice leads to a deep state of relaxation, or perhaps some great ideas will come into your head. You may find that fears dissolve or you may even hear the 'whisperings of the inner voice'. Either way, the benefits of regular meditation practice are often very powerful.

Conscious breathing can be practiced throughout the day. Taking a 'firm but fair' inhalation and then relaxing completely on the exhalation, and being aware that you are a living, breathing being is known as 'conscious circular breathing' and in its own way is a kind of meditation. I guess that adepts breathe in this way all the time. Check yourself periodically through the day, are you on 'auto pilot' or are you 'conscious'. You may find that your breathing is irregular and short, in which case it will be impossible to attain any kind of 'peace' or 'equanimity of mind'. If you notice this, start the conscious breathing and continue with your day.

If you want to practice meditation sitting upright in a chair or cross-legged, you may want to create a focus - perhaps a single candle on a small table or some pictures or icons of your chosen god/s. Sitting in the same place at the same time every day, even if just for 5 minutes, is an excellent way to get used to the benefits of meditation. The subconscious mind will start to recognize this daily meditation pattern and a sense of calm throughout the day will often occur relatively quickly.

Some other tips regarding meditation include:

> Avoid practicing when you are full of food or if you need the urgency to go to the toilet.

> If someone or something disturbs you, treat it as part of the practice and carry on regardless of whatever interruption you face.

> Meditate on you own (as most people prefer) or in a group (which can often lead to a more powerful experience)

> Try to eat natural foods generally, as a junk food diet is not good for your mind

See the Appendices section to read what is written in the Bhagavad Gita about meditation.

JYOTI (LIGHT) MEDITATION

Perhaps the most important of all the various meditations, Jyoti meditation is taught by Sathya Sai Baba as well as numerous other spiritual teachers and yogis. Of it he says:

'Have a lamp with a bright steady flame or a candle before you. Sit in the padmasana (cross legged) posture or any other comfortable asana in front of the flame. Look at the flame steadily. Then closing your eyes, try to feel the flame inside you, between your eye brows. From there let it descend down into the lotus of your heart, in the centre of the chest, illuminating the path.

When it enters the heart, imagine that the petals of the lotus bud open out, one by one, bathing every thought, feeling, emotion and impulse in the light and so removing darkness there. There is no space now for darkness to take refuge. It has to flee before the flame.

Imagine that the light becomes wider, bigger and brighter. Let it pervade the limbs; now these limbs can never more deal in dark, suspicious and wicked activities. These have become instruments of light and love.

Let the light reach up to the tongue and falsehood, slander and spite vanish from it. Let it rise up to the eyes and the ears and destroy all the dark desires therein. Let your head be surcharged with light and all the wicked thoughts flee therefrom, for these are the denizens of darkness. Imagine that light in you more and more intensely and it will become so. Let it shine all around you and let it spread from you in ever widening circles, taking in your loved ones, your kith and kin, your friends and companions, your enemies and rivals, strangers, all living beings, the entire world. Stay on in that thrill of witnessing light. If you are adoring God in any form, now try to visualise that form in the all pervasive light, for light is God and God is light.'

Benefits of regular yoga practice

PHYSIOLOGICAL

> Stable autonomic nervous system equilibrium
> Pulse rate decreases
> Respiratory rate decreases
> Blood Pressure decreases
> Galvanic Skin Response (GSR) increases
> EEG - alpha waves increase (theta, delta, and beta waves also increase during various stages of meditation)
> EMG activity decreases
> Cardiovascular efficiency increases
> Respiratory efficiency increases
> Gastrointestinal function normalizes
> Endocrine function normalizes
> Excretory functions improve
> Musculoskeletal flexibility and joint range of motion increase

➢ Breath-holding time increases

➢ Joint range of motion increase

➢ Grip strength increases

➢ Eye-hand coordination improves

➢ Dexterity skills improve

➢ Reaction time improves

➢ Posture improves

➢ Strength and resiliency increase

➢ Endurance increases

➢ Energy level increases

➢ Weight normalizes

➢ Sleep improves

➢ Immunity increases

➢ Pain decreases

➢ Steadiness improves

➢ Depth perception improves

➢ Balance improves

➢ Integrated functioning of body parts improves

PSYCHOLOGICAL

➢ Somatic and kinaesthetic awareness increase

➢ Mood improves and subjective well-being increases

➢ Self-acceptance and self-actualisation increase

➢ Social adjustment increases

➢ Anxiety and Depression decrease

➢ Hostility decreases

➢ Concentration improves

- Memory improves
- Attention improves
- Learning efficiency improves
- Mood improves
- Self-actualisation increase
- Social skills increase
- Well-being increases
- Self-acceptance increase
- Attention improves
- Concentration improves
- Memory improves
- Learning efficiency improves
- Symbol coding improves
- Depth perception improves
- Flicker fusion frequency improves

YOGA BENEFITS VERSUS SPORT EXERCISE BENEFITS

Yoga benefits

- Parasympathetic Nervous System dominates
- Sub cortical regions of brain dominate
- Slow dynamic and static movements
- Normalization of muscle tone
- Low risk of injuring muscles and ligaments
- Low caloric consumption
- Effort is minimized, relaxed

> ➤ Energizing (breathing is natural or controlled)
> ➤ Balanced activity of opposing muscle groups
> ➤ Non-competitive, process-oriented
> ➤ Awareness is internal (focus is on breath and the infinite)
> ➤ Limitless possibilities for growth in self-awareness

Sport exercise drawbacks

> ➤ Sympathetic Nervous System dominates
> ➤ Cortical regions of brain dominate
> ➤ Rapid forceful movements
> ➤ Increased muscle tension
> ➤ Higher risk of injury
> ➤ Moderate to high caloric consumption
> ➤ Effort is maximized
> ➤ Fatiguing (breathing is taxed)
> ➤ Imbalance activity of opposing groups
> ➤ Competitive, goal-oriented
> ➤ Awareness is external (focus is on reaching the toes, reaching the finish line, etc.

Below is a flyer, I once made promoting yoga:

Simply put, Yoga works...

It makes you feel lighter, healthier...Yoga is the ultimate self-improvement system. It is a way of living and experiencing a really good life, not just a technique or daily exercise routine. Yoga makes us stronger in body, mind and in spirit...There is an abundance of research that shows Yoga helps manage or control:

Anxiety, Asthma, Stress, Heart Disease, Insomnia, Back Pain, Arthritis, Carpel Tunnel Syndrome, Depression, Menopausal Symptoms, Headaches (including Migraines Fibromyalgia), Blood Pressure, Chronic Fatigue Syndrome, Addictions, Diabetes, Multiple Sclerosis and Epilepsy...

Yoga also:

Improves muscle tone, flexibility, strength and stamina

Reduces tension

Improves self esteem

Boosts concentration and creativity levels

Lowers fat

Aids circulation

Stimulates the immune system

Creates a sense of calmness and well-being

Over time, with Yoga, muscle tone and flexibility improve. These changes in the physical body usually result in an increase in energy, they improve overall general health and lead the way towards reconnecting with yourself.

Yoga is a process through which we can learn to accept and enjoy who we are - just as we are.

Nasal cleansing (Neti)

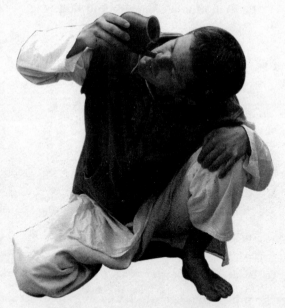

Fig. 6.21 Nasal Cleansing (Neti)

The 'Neti' is an ancient Indian yoga technique that literally means 'water cleansing'. The nasal cavity is rinsed with saline water using a neti pot and the technique is starting to be recognized by science under the term nasal irrigation.

The practice of neti, though relatively unknown to western culture, is a common practice in parts of India and other areas in southeast Asia. When dealing with problems of congestion it can be performed up to three times a day and has been shown to speed up the healing process for common colds.

Procedure

A typical method utilizes an isotonic saline solution. This matches roughly the concentration of salt found in the blood. Use 1/4 teaspoon of real, unadulterated salt for every 1/4 litre of water. The solution is then heated to approximately the temperature as the blood in the body (cold water can be added to boiled water to reach the desired temperature). Make sure the salt is thoroughly dissolved by stirring. Check the temperature of the water by pouring a little of it over the back of your hand.

The technique has three stages:

> Over a sink, bathtub, or outdoors on the ground, the head is held with the forehead and chin at roughly the same level facing downward.

> The spout is then placed in one nostril and then that same nostril is tilted upward and along with the neti pot to begin pouring the water into that nostril.

> Breathing is continued through the mouth. The water flows down and out the lower nostril.

Half of the solution is used for each side. If the water flows freely then it can be done in two passes, one for each side. If the water seems to be blocked, switching back and forth several times may help.

Once the neti has been performed, it is important to eliminate any remaining water from the nose. Bend over and breathe quick breaths out the nose in quick repetition. It is important not to close off one nostril or squeeze the nose in any way as this may cause water to be forced into areas that do not dry easily and may cause infection such as in the ear canal. A tissue may be used but is just held lightly surrounding the nose. Never blow out too hard.

If the nasal cavity is particularly dirty, there may be stinging sensation for a small time as the water passes through, this is nothing to worry about.

Benefits

> Reduction of allergy problems

> Improvement to breathing

> Elimination of post-nasal drip

> Elimination of sinusitis or chronic sinus infections

> Common colds are either avoided or the duration greatly shortened

> General improvement to sinus health

> Vision is clearer. Neti will actually clean the tear ducts enabling better cleaning and moistening of the eyes

> Improved sense of smell

> Improved sense of taste

> Deeper and more relaxed breathing

> Helps with breathing exercises (especially nadi shodhana)

The practice of pranayama is greatly enhanced by the practice of neti since many of them involve deep breathing through the nostrils.

Cautions

Some people may have hardened blockages. These may be eliminated gradually over several attempts but in case it is due to a deviated septum a minor surgery may be needed.

Attimes there might be burning or irritation of the nasal lining. This is why it is crucial to get the right temperature and salinity and to test it by taking a sip first.

A person may feel sharp pains due to pressure on the sinuses. They should stop immediately and consult a healthcare professional.

If you experience ear discomfort when performing neti, you should be sure to blow the nose more gently after the wash. If the problem persists, the openings of their eustachian tubes may be particularly wide and you may need to discontinue the practice.

Hand positions (Mudra)

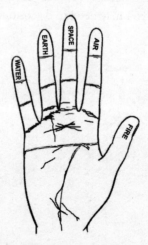

Fig. 6.22 Hand Mudra showing five elements

If you look closely the pictures of Hindu gods, you may well find that they are holding their fingers and thumbs in specific hand positions. These hand positions are known as 'mudras' and they are an integral part of yoga, with numerous health benefits for those who take the time to practice them.

What most yoga books fail to tell readers is how mudras actually work, so to begin with I'll explore some of the 'mechanics' behind ayurveda, yoga and mudras.

FIVE ELEMENTS AND THREE HUMOURS

As with ancient Chinese philosophy, there are five elements, which serve a critical and specific function within the body. These five elements are commonly known as space, air, water, fire and earth.

Air

All movements in the body are affected by air, so this element is of movement. This includes movement of thoughts, emotions and bioelectricity. It also regulates the sense of touch and hence the skin.

Space

Interactive, it manifests in the body cavities (e.g. the ear cavity). Its role is to create space in the body to facilitate the functions of the other elements.

Fire

Controls body temperature and metabolism. It causes thirst, hunger, digestion and assimilation. It also relates to vision and hence the eyes.

Water

Is the constituent of protoplasm, blood, tears, sweat, urine, semen, cerebrospinal fluid and fat. It also relates to taste and hence the tongue.

Earth

Is responsible for body mass and is the constituent of skin, hair, nails, bones, cartilage, muscles etc. Earth is associated with smell and hence the nose.

KAPHA, PITTA AND VATA

According to the ayurvedic and Chinese healthcare systems, health results from a balance (or homeostasis) of these five elements. Mudra yoga works well because each of the four fingers and the thumb corresponds to the five elements (see picture above). Ayurveda focuses on the three humours of the body; kapha, pitta and vata. These humours also correspond to the five elements, as shown below.

Element	Corresponding humour
Air	vata
Space	vata
Fire	pitta
Water	pitta
Earth	kapha

In a typical Ayurvedic consultation, the patient will be classified according to the balance of their three humours, usually with one humour being predominant. Without going into too much detail, an example of an 'overly vata' constitution would be a patient with too much 'air headedness', shallow breathing and anxiety, whereas an example of someone being 'overly kapha' would be too much excess weight, a lack-lustre approach to life and suffering from a greedy disposition. Balance is the key and most therapeutic systems agree.

Here's how the mudras work. The thumb acts as the battery charger with the 'fire' emanating from it's tip. When the tip of the thumb touches the tip of any of the fingers, it incrementally increases the corresponding element/humour. For instance, when the index finger is touched to the thumb (as in Gyan mudra), it leads to an increase of air/vata in the body (amongst other effects). However, when the little finger tip is touched by the thumb, it leads to an increase of the water element/pitta.

To decrease any particular element/humour, simply place the finger at the base of the thumb where it meets the palm.

All that is left to do, is to know which particular humour/element you need to focus on and increase or decrease it by steadily applying the correct mudra.

Mudras can be practiced in any number of different places and situations, for example:

- On the bus
- When walking
- Lying in bed
- Watching the TV
- During a yoga session

PRACTICAL TIPS

- Only a light contact between the thumb and finger is necessary.
- It doesn't matter if the other fingers are relaxed or tensed.
- It is more effective to do mudras using both hands simultaneously.
- Better results accompany a calm mind and steady, relaxed breathing pattern.
- A rubber band or some tape can be used to hold the chosen finger/s and thumb together.
- Thirty minutes to an hour per day is recommended. This can be done all in one go or in blocks of say, fifteen minutes.

GYAN MUDRA

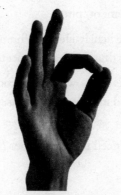

Fig. 6.23 Gyan Mudra

Index finger touches thumb tip.

Effects

➢ Completes the bio-electro-magnetic circuitry of the body (thumb = positive energy; index finger = negative energy).

➢ Empowerment of mind, emotions, nervous system, bioelectricity, endocrine glands, muscles, vocal chords and heart.

PRAN MUDRA

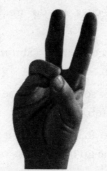

Fig. 6.24 Pran Mudra

Third finger and little finger tips touch the thumb tip.

Effects

- ➤ Increases vitality
- ➤ Reduces fatigue / nervousness
- ➤ Improves vision
- ➤ Increases will power and assertiveness & self-confidence

(Clear eyes are also a sign of a mental outlook emphasizing clarity and a clear mind, which means clearly structured thoughts and ideas).

APAN MUDRA

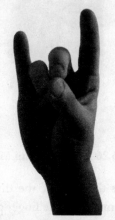

Fig. 6.25 Apan Mudra

Second and third finger tips touch the thumb.

Effects

- ➤ Supports the removal of waste materials and toxins from the body.
- ➤ Helps to overcome urinary problems.

> Stimulates the liver and gallbladder.

> Has a balancing effect on the mind.

> Promotes patience, serenity, confidence, inner balance, and harmony.

A balanced, calm mind is closely connected with a well-functioning liver.

MRITSANJEEVINI MUDRA

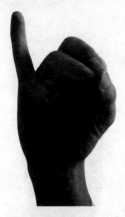

Fig. 6.26 Mritsanjeevini Mudra

Index finger tip presses the base of the thumb. Second and third fingertips touch the thumb tip. Little finger points away.

Effect

> Strengthens the heart (it is said that this mudra can avert a heart attack, if it is performed within a couple of seconds).

LINGA MUDRA

Palms are clasped tightly together with one thumb sticking upward.

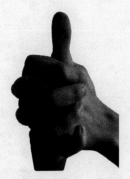

Fig. 6.27 Linga Mudra

Effects

- ➤ Strengthens the respiratory tract.
- ➤ Loosens mucus that has collected in the lungs.
- ➤ Increases the body temperature.
- ➤ Stimulates the digestive system.
- ➤ Can help to lose excess weight.

Chi Kung

*'The softest thing in the universe.
Overcomes the hardest thing in the universe.
That without substance can enter where there is no room.
Hence I know the value of non-action.
Teaching without words and work without doing.
Are understood by very few.'*

- Lao Tse

Chi kung is an ancient system of health and healing that harnesses the natural, universal chi energy. Chi kung can be defined as:

'Vital energy, biological energy or life force that is inherent in all things.'

It is the same force that the Yoga systems call 'prana' and without it life cannot exist. Kung can be translated as:

'Practice, cultivate or refine.'

So chi kung can be loosely translated as 'energy practice'. As one of the five pillars of traditional Chinese medicine, chi kung is practiced daily by millions of Chinese people as well as a growing number in the west. The simple and peaceful movements have proved popular amongst all age groups and the benefits are well worth the time and effort spent to learn the basics. The other three pillars of traditional Chinese medicine are acupuncture, massage and herbal remedies. Of these, chi kung is the one that can be most easily self-learned and is thought to be the mother of Chinese healing.

By increasing and facilitating the flow of chi in and around the body, disease can be countered and replaced with vitality and a sense of equilibrium. The specific movements, breaths and postures give rise to increased levels of oxygen to the tissues, enhances the elimination of waste products through the lymphatic system and catapults a spontaneous balancing and enhancing of the natural healing capacities within us.

There are hundreds of different varieties of chi kung, each focusing on a specific aspect of human potential. Some are elaborate, some very simple, some gentle and some very hard. In the same way that one chi kung master could use his internal forces to help heal someone; another could use those same forces to perform amazing feats of mind over matter. The following exercises are an excellent introduction to chi kung and are particularly effective as techniques that anyone can fairly easily learn and safely practice without a competent teacher. As with yoga, it is very important to be patient and persistent when practicing, setting aside a certain time each day if possible. Diligently work through the steps and get used to the exercises. In time, the wonderfully cumulative effects will start to emerge as chi levels in the body increase.

WU CHI

The words 'Wu' and 'Chi' mean:

Wu = absence, negation or nothingness.

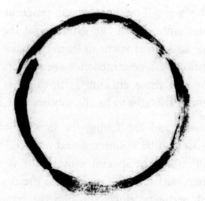

Fig. 6.28 Chi Energy Circle

Chi = Highest or ultimate (not to be confused with the 'Chi' that refers to life force.)

Therefore Wu Chi can be defined as:

'Ultimate state of nothingness'.

Wu chi is symbolised by the empty circle, which represents the state of pure openness. The taoists gave the name wu chi to the state of total emptiness that existed before the universe became manifest. The concept of time (a relative concept) did not exist in this primordial state because there was no reference point to measure the time form.

The wu chi stance develops and initiates postural awareness. In the Yoga Chi Kung syllabus, it is often adopted before and after the various chi kung exercises. In many ways, it is a 'standing meditation' position that allows a free-flow of energy around the relaxed, upright body.

Technique

Stand on the feet, shoulder width apart in the usual way. Keeping the

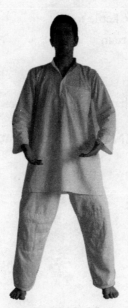

Fig. 6.29 Wu Chi Stance

spine straight, imagine the top of the spine is being pulled up to the sky whilst the base of the spine is being pulled towards to the earth. This has the effect of very gently pulling each vertebra apart which releases tension in the discs and frees up the flow of chi energy.

Relax the shoulders and hold the arms out slightly as shown in the diagram above.

As with all chi kung exercises, keep reminding yourself to relax the abdominal muscles and breathe in the correct way. The area just below the naval is known as the lower 'tan tien'. It is the body's centre of gravity and the main area for storing chi energy.

The wu chi stance is very simple and very powerful. If performed correctly, the whole body will feel pleasantly warm, energised and relaxed. The wu chi position can be practiced almost anywhere, anytime:

> ➤ Waiting for the kettle to boil
> ➤ Standing on a train
> ➤ Watching TV
> ➤ Looking out to sea
> ➤ Any time you have a minute to spare

SPINE ALIGNMENT AGAINST A WALL

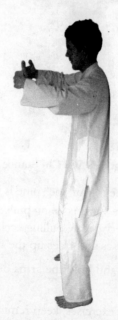

Fig. 6.30 Spine alignment against a wall

This is a simple and powerful exercise to teach your body how to stand correctly, after a few minutes; it leads to the release of chi energy.

Take shoes off and find any free area of wall. Place the feet 2 inches from the wall and shoulder width apart (feet parallel).

Place the arms out in front of you as in position 2 of Zhan Zhuang (as if you are holding a large beach ball against your chest).

Gently push two spinal vertebrae against the wall, the one that sticks out slightly between the hips area and the one that is located directly between the shoulder blades.

Relax the soles of the feet and focus on circular breathing.

CARRYING THE MOON

Stand with the feet parallel and keep shoulder width apart approximately. Exhale as you slowly and gently bend down until the arms are hanging down towards the feet.

Inhale as you slowly raise the arms above the head in a big arc in front of the body until they are above the head, keeping the palms facing skyward. Stretch the arms straight and push the palms up.

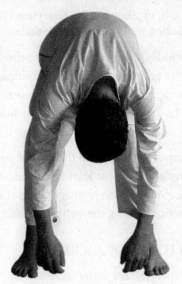

Fig. 6.31 (a)

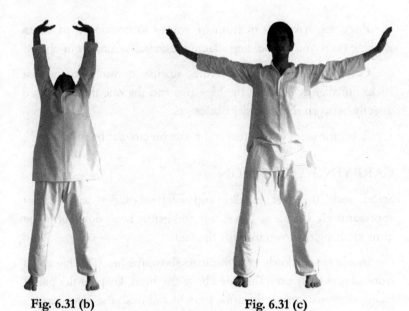

Fig. 6.31 (b)   **Fig. 6.31 (c)**

**Fig. 6.31 (a, b, c) Showing the Carrying The Moon
during inhalation and exhalation**

Exhale as you slowly lower the arms out to the sides of the body in a big arc, until the palms are down by the side of the thighs. As the arms come down, visualise and feel the lowering of the energy, down through the body; from the crown of the head to the base of the torso, down through the legs and into the earth.

Take a breath or two, standing in the wu chi position. Relax and start the process again. Repeat at least five times. I particularly like this exercise as it begins to feel very invigorating after a few minutes. The longer the practice session, the better the feeling!

STANDING STILL LIKE A TREE

This simple yet powerful chi kung exercise has been used as a supplementary form of healing in Chinese hospitals since the 1950's.

314

As well as a means to attain excellent health and longevity, it is also a way to steadily develop internal chi energy in a highly pronounced way. 'Standing still like a tree' (or 'zhan zhuang' – roughly pronounced as 'chan chong') is one of the key exercises of chi kung.

I started practicing zhan zhuang as a boy and was quite taken by the effect it had on me. After about twenty minutes of practice, I would feel surges of electricity darting around my body, which was an enjoyable and energising experience. The various positions are easy to learn, however it takes dedication and perseverance to keep practicing daily and reap the deeper benefits.

The positions work for the muscles in the arms and on the legs that don't usually get used so much in daily life, so it can be tough in the beginning. Once the muscles develop strength, the exercise becomes more easy and pleasurable to perform.

Zhan zhuang training is ideally suited for correcting problems stemming from the imbalance between phasic muscles and postural muscles. The emphasis on tranquillity is very beneficial in any stress-related problems and the training method of slow and careful movements improves co-ordination and balance. It is an excellent method of regulating one's metabolism and sleep pattern.

In the beginning, hold each of the positions for only two minutes or so and incrementally build up the duration from there onwards. Holding each position comfortably for five minutes can be seen as intermediate level and comfortably holding each position for ten minutes or more can be seen as more advanced practice.

Position 1: Chi Storage Position

Palms crossed over each other (right over left for men and left over right for women) over the 'tan tien', two inches below the naval. Visualise a fire of chi burning in this point and radiating the heat throughout the whole body.

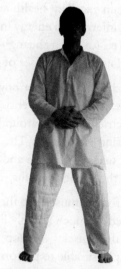

Fig. 6.32 (a) Chi storage position

Position 2: Holding the beach ball to the chest

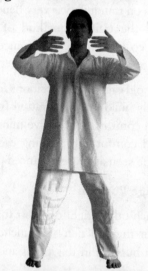

Fig. 6.32 (b) Holding the beach ball to the chest

Slowly raise your arms up as if holding a large beach ball. Notice any bio-electro-magnetic changes in your body, relax the shoulders and try to relax those muscles in the arms that don't need tensing.

Position 3: Marriage of heaven and earth

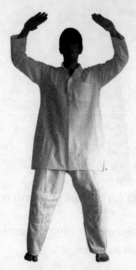

Fig. 6.32 (c) Marriage of heaven and earth

Slowly raise arms to just above the head and turn palms outward. Visualise cosmic energy coming in through the palms and earth energy coming in through the feet. Feel the chi energy in your body merging and blending with the chi energy with both the heavenly and earthly realms.

Position 4: Absorbing Earth energy

Slowly lower the arms to the side of the body and turn the palms to face downward. Visualise earth chi coming in through the soles of the feet and the palms.

317

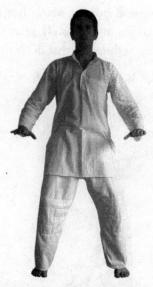

Fig. 6.32 (d) Absorbing earth energy

Return to the chi storage position to finish. Hold each position for between one and ten minutes.

CHI BALL CULTIVATION

From the sitting position or standing wu chi position, gently raise the right hand so it is at the height of your chest with the palm open and facing downwards. The left hand is at the level of the abdomen with the palm open and facing upwards.

Slowly turn the body to the left (the fingers of the upper hand always point in the direction the body is turning). The hands keep the position they are in and move with the body.

When you are facing towards the left, slowly lower and turn the right hand whilst rising and turning the left hand so their positions are reversed.

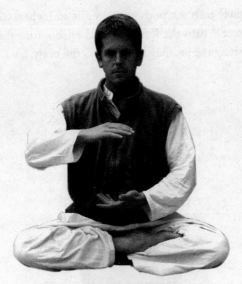

Fig. 6.33 (a) Chi Ball Cultivation

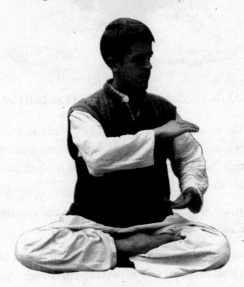

Fig. 6.33 (b)

Now slowly turn the body to the right and when you are facing the right, lower / turn the left hand and raise / turn the right hand before beginning the journey back across the body, back towards the right.

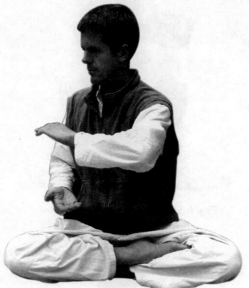

Fig. 6.33 (c)

Fig. 6.33 (b, c) Showing variations in Chi Ball Cultivation

At all times, keep the hands equally distant apart, as if you are holding a ball of energy that must not be dropped. A short stick (approximately 30cm) can be held between the palms of each hand to ensure that they stay in the right place.

Concentrate on gentle circular breathing and visualise the energy ball at all times.

This exercise can be practiced anytime you have a few moments to spare and is an excellent way to develop chi energy whilst focussing and calming the mind.

When practicing chi kung exercises, always remember the following points:

> Relax the soles of the feet, remembering the three points where the weight of the body should be distributed.

> Relax the shoulders. Avoid the temptation to hunch them slightly.

> Breath in a calm and steady way.

> Relax the facial muscles and all other muscles that do not need to be tensed in order to hold each position.

> Focus on feeling the different parts of the body. For instance, as you lower the arms into the 'absorbing earth energy' position, try focussing on the soles of your feet for while. Then focus on the palms of the hands.

> Generally keep the neck straight and chin slightly down.

> Keep the abdominal muscles relaxed.

> Smile inwardly.

THE INNER SMILE

The Inner Smile refers to the simple and essential practice of harnessing the power of the smile (happiness and joy) and allowing that power to permeate the whole of the body. One method is to cast your mind back to an experience when you were genuinely happy and smiling. Then you imagine that energy is flowing into all the internal organs and around the body. It is not necessary for the mouth to be grinning (although it is not a bad thing if it is) as long as the feeling of happiness and joy is present. The inner smile should be practiced as often as possible, especially during internal exercises.

Some things I might think about to feel happy:

Concerning the practice of the Inner Smile, chi kung master

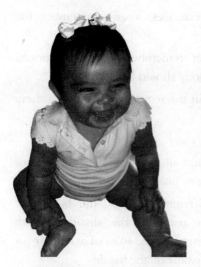 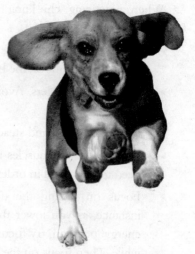

Fig. 6.34 (a) A baby, full of joy
and love

Fig. 6.34 (b) A dog, also full
of joy and love

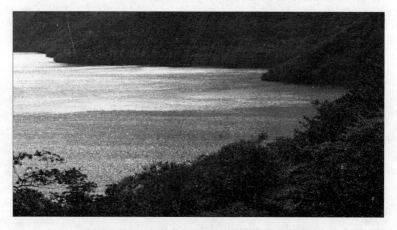

Fig. 6.34 (c) A beautiful summer morning

Fig. 6.34 (a, b, c) Few examples of Inner smile

Mantak Chia says:

In ancient China, the Taoists taught that a constant inner smile, a smile to oneself, insured health, happiness and longevity. Why? Smiling to yourself is like basking in love: you become your own best friend. Living with an inner smile is to live in harmony with yourself...

'As a formal practice, the energy of the Inner Smile can be consciously directed downward into the heart, the belly, the liver, the stomach and to other digestive organs; to the bones, blood, nervous system ... to the whole of the body ... in directed flows through particular parts of the body or as a global radiating whole. You can apply these flows intuitively while sitting quietly.'

Chi energy can be negative as well as positive. Damaging emotions are a form of chi that can arise from energetic blockages in the body. Outbursts of anger and frustration or episodes of fear, loneliness or confusion can also cause blockages in a specific organ or its associated channel of energy. For instance, frustration is said to be the primary cause of liver chi stagnation, so it can work both ways; blockages cause negative emotions and vice-versa. This downward cycle can be reversed by the simple practice of the inner smile.

A smile is a powerful tool for communication – smile and the world smiles with you. A genuine smile gives a message of:

> Acceptance

> Love

> Understanding

> Appreciation

> Safety

It activates our parasympathetic nervous system's 'relaxation response', which in turn produces a variety of changes in our:

> ➤ Endocrine glands
> ➤ Nervous system
> ➤ Muscles
> ➤ Respiratory tract
> ➤ Digestive system

So as well as being a fine way to communicate with others, a smile is also a healing tool in communicating with ourselves.

The more you practice the inner smile, the easier it will become to achieve a wholesome, healthy and joyous state of being.

The Five Tibetan Rites

In 1985 a book called 'The Ancient Secret of the Fountain of Youth' by Peter Kelder was published which for the first time fully described a simple exercise program for 'youthing'. These exercises are used by Tibetan monks to live long, vibrant and healthy lives. The book also states that many have lived longer than most can imagine by following the program often called 'The Five Tibetan Rites'.

In the 'Ancient Secret of the Fountain of Youth: Book 2' (a companion to Kelder's original book) benefits were listed such as:

> Looking much younger

> Sleeping soundly

> Waking up feeling refreshed and energetic

> Release from serious medical problems including difficulties with the spine

> Relief from problems with joints

> Release from pain

> Better memory

> Relief from Arthritis

> Weight loss

> Improved vision

> 'Youthing' instead of aging

> Greatly improved physical strength

> Endurance and vigour

> Improved emotional and mental health

> Enhanced sense of well-being and harmony

> Very high overall energy

Most practitioners of the Five Tibetan Rites share the view that they represent a system of exercise that affects the body, emotions and mind. The Tibetans claim that these exercises activate and stimulate the seven key charkas (the major energy vortexes that form the underlying basis of the physical human being); that in turn stimulate all the glands of the endocrine system. The endocrine system is responsible for the body's overall functioning and aging process. This means that the Five Tibetan Rites affect the functioning of all the organs and systems.

The rugged mountainous conditions these monks live in may well account for their particular emphasis on vigour. Many of the yoga exercises and practices being taught in the western world today are very new. It is very important to do the Rites exactly as they are presented without altering the form or sequence.

Caution: Spinning and stretching through the following exercises can aggravate certain health conditions such as any type of heart problem, multiple sclerosis, Parkinson's disease, severe arthritis of the spine, uncontrolled high blood pressure, a hyperthyroid condition or vertigo. The problems may also be caused if you are taking drugs that cause dizziness. Please consult a competent healthcare practitioner prior to beginning these exercises if you have any health issues or any other concerns.

Rite 1

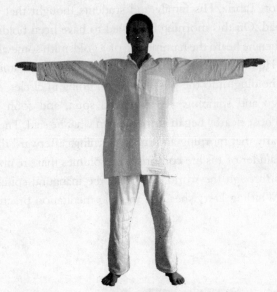

Fig. 6.35 Rite 1

Stand erect with arms outstretched horizontal to the floor, palms facing down. Your arms should be in line with your shoulders. Spin around clockwise until you become slightly dizzy. Each 360-degree rotation should take about three seconds. Gradually increase from 3 to 21 spins as you get more used to it. Each revolution should take between one to two seconds.

Inhale and exhale deeply as you spin.

A note on Rumi

Rumi was the original Whirling Dervish. One account of Rumi's first whirling experience tells us that he was standing in the courtyard outside his family home early one morning. It had been two years since he had last spoken, having fallen into silence after the disappearance and presumed death of his beloved spiritual teacher and friend, Shams of Tabriz. His family and students thought that Rumi had gone mad. On this morning he is said to have been holding onto a post, when he heard the hammering of a goldsmith somewhere in the village. He began moving his feet to the beat of the hammer. Since he was holding onto the post, he began going in circles, eventually, letting go and spinning. He spun and spun, and soon started to speak. Those nearby began writing down what he said. The words he spoke early that morning and most mornings afterward throughout the remainder of his life comprise the volumes that are now read by millions through the world. This was the inaugural spin, the birth of the Whirling Dervishes, the moving meditation practice of the Sufis.

Rite 2

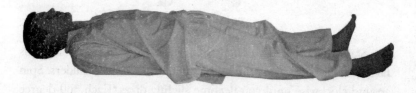

Fig. 6.36 (a) Rite 2

Lie flat on the floor; face up. Fully extend your arms along your sides and place the palms of your hands against the floor, keeping fingers close together. Then raise your head off the floor tucking your chin into your chest.

As you do this, lift your legs, knees straight, into a vertical

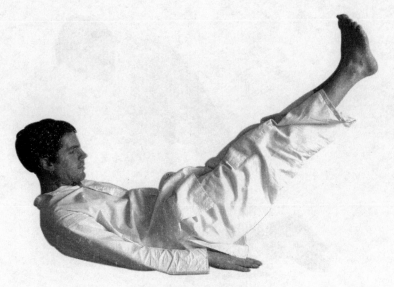

Fig. 6.36 (b) Rite 2

position. If possible, extend the legs over the body towards your head. Do not let the knees bend. Then slowly lower the legs and head to the floor, always keeping the knees straight. Allow the muscles to relax, and repeat.

Breathe in deeply as you lift your head and legs and exhale as you lower your head and legs.

Rite 3

Kneel on the floor with the body erect. The hands should be placed on the backs of your thigh muscles. Incline the head and neck forward, tucking your chin in against your chest. Then throw the head and neck backward, arching the spine. Your toes should be curled under through this exercise. As you arch, you will brace your arms and hands against the thighs for support. After the arching, return your body to an erect position and begin the rite all over again.

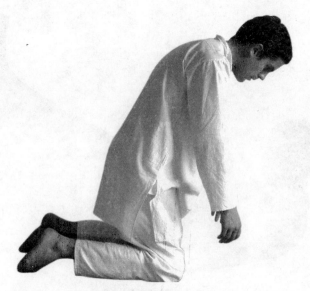

Fig. 6.37 (a) Rite 3

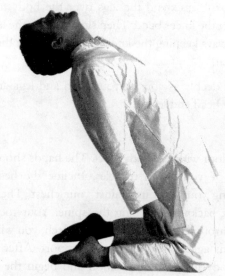

Fig. 6.37 (b) Rite 3

Inhale as you arch the spine and exhale as you return to an erect position.

Rite 4

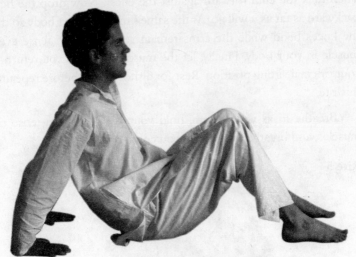

Fig. 6.38 (a) Rite 4

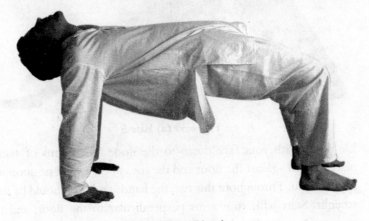

Fig. 6.38 (b) Rite 4

Sit down on the floor with your legs straight out in front of you and your feet shoulder width apart. With the trunk of the body erect, place the palms of your hands on the floor alongside your buttocks. Then tuck the chin forward against the chest. Now drop the head backward as far as it will go. At the same time raise your body so that the knees bend while the arms remain straight. Then tense every muscle in your body. Finally, let the muscles relax as you return to your original sitting position. Rest for a short while before repeating this rite.

Breathe in as you rise up, hold your breath as you tense the muscles, and breathe out fully as you come down.

Rite 5

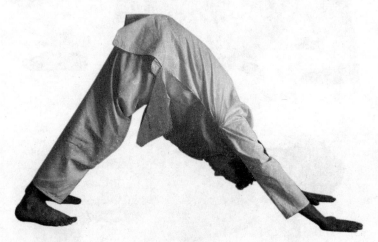

Fig. 6.39 (a) Rite 5

Lie down with your face down to the floor. The palms of hands placed down against the floor and the toes in the flexed position will support you. Throughout this rite, the hands and feet should be kept straight. Start with your arms perpendicular to the floor, and the spine arched, so that the body is in a sagging position. Now throw

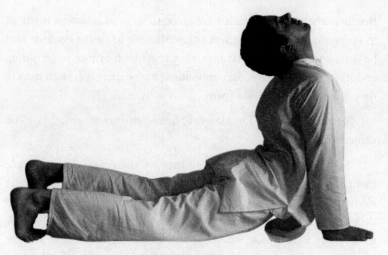

Fig. 6.39 (b) Rite 5

the head back as far as possible with the bending at the hips, bring the body up into an inverted 'V'. At the same time, bring the chin forward, tucking it against the chest.

Breathe in deeply as you raise the body, and exhale fully as you lower the body.

SUNLIGHT

Essential to health, the sun and its rays are essential for life on Earth. Practicing exercises, walking, sitting and lying under the sun is an integral part of the Five Point Plan and is recommended for people of all ages.

In his book 'Human Culture and Cure', Dr. G D Babbit writes:

'There is a vast array of forces of every kind, including iron, magnesium, sodium, carbon, and of other elements conveyed by the sunlight; but why not take these elements in their ordinary form from our drugstores, and not go to the trouble of taking sun-baths?

333

Because when these elements are given to us in so refined a form, as to come directly from the sun as an ether, or to float skywards and be driven to us by the solar rays, they must be far more penetrating, enduring, safe, pleasant, and upbuilding to the mental system than if they were used in a crude form.'

Natural Hygienist Dr. Herbert Shelton throws more light on the subject:

'Sunlight dominates the chemistry of the blood. On a simple natural diet, with sufficient sunlight, the blood will contain the elements it requires for life and growth. Pills, capsules, and liquid drugs of lime, iron, sulphur, phosphorus, etc are of no earthly value to the body, well or sick, whether given in the sun or out of it. Nature Curists have for years advocated eating sun-cooked foods. 'Eat the sun's rays' was an expression with them. Recent experiments have shown that their instincts and reason had not led them astray: Plants or animals raised in the sun have shown better health and more food value. Milk from 'sun-fed' animals contains more vitamins.'

He further elucidates this by adding:

'A vitamin is probably not something different from the rest of the food. It is probably not a distinct chemical substance, but merely a peculiar grouping brought about the action of the sun's rays, which renders the food, or some part of it, more easily assimilated and used by the body.'

This way of perceiving what a vitamin really is, seems to reflect both yoga and chi kung's philosophical basis that 'everything is a frequency, even what appears to be solid matter'. Both disciplines have adepts who are capable of living perfectly healthily without the need for food or water; they simply live off fresh air and sunlight. In the yogic tradition this skill is called 'pranic nourishment' and in the chi kung tradition it is called 'bigu'. Adepts claim that they absorb and utilise the energies of sun and air in much the same way that a plant does through photosynthesis.

In his excellent paper 'Heliotherapy & Practice of Sunbathing' John Fielder ends his section 'Heliotherapy and health' with the following two postulates:

1. In the case of the so-called bactericidal properties of sunlight, that what we actually are observing is the overall changing of the environmental conditions bringing about a situation whereby the need or necessity of bacteriological or virological action is no longer required. The bacteria or virus, as the case may be, then either die, or leave, or a Bechamp suggests, regain their former condition as microzyma.

2. In the case of the increased white blood cells, particularly in the lymphocytes, that this phenomena has particularly to do with the increased metabolism with its concurrent increase in the elimination of accumulated toxic waste matter, which manifests in the above-mentioned way.

Sunlight is essential for all-round physical fitness. Dr. Kime says:

Before the time of Christ, men such as Herodotus and Antyllus believed in the beneficial effects of the sunlight in promoting physical fitness. They believed that, 'The sun feeds the muscles.' The Romans made use of the sun for training their gladiators, for they knew that sunlight seemed to strengthen and enlarge the muscles.

Natural Hygienist Dr. James Jackson writes in 'The Hygienic System' that:

'A man who lives out in the sunlight will grow thin in the flesh but full in the nerve. His muscles will diminish, but as they diminish his nerves become increased in size and strengthened, and their action on the muscles is such as to decidedly strengthen these; so that when one comes to look at him and judge of his strength by his apparent bulk, if he does not understand and fully appreciate the effect of living largely in the sunlight, he will greatly misjudge his muscular abilities.'

The suns rays increase oxygen in the tissues thus helping with fatigue problems and increasing the body's endurance to cope with day-to-day life and prevent / overcome health problems.

Sunbathing tips

> If you are unused to being out in the sun, proceed with caution and come into the shade as soon as you start to feel overheated. Increase the amount of time spent in the sun gently and incrementally.

> Morning sunbathing is recommended because the ultraviolet rays predominate in the morning.

> The palms of the hands and soles of the feet contain a vast amount of nerve endings, so make sure that some sunlight reaches these parts of the body.

> Receiving sunlight through a glass or plastic window will not give the health benefits of direct sunlight.

> Both the aged and those who are sick are far more sensitive to the sun's rays and must take greater care than younger / healthier people.

> Blond and red haired people need less sunlight than dark haired people because the light can pass through light skin more readily than through darker skin.

> The strength of the sun's rays increases with elevation, so be careful not to burn when sunbathing at the high altitude.

> Always lie with the head away from the sun and cover the scalp, if you are bald.

➢ Avoid wearing sunglasses because sunlight is beneficial for the vision (contrary to popular opinion).

➢ Avoid wearing suntan and sunscreen lotions as their chemicals may well cause the very conditions that they claim to protect against.

Summary

Enjoying regular exercise (both internal and external) is an important part of staying healthy and happy. Make your commitment to exercise a long term one and remember that a few minutes practice each day is much better than two hours a day and then nothing for two weeks. Set aside a certain time of the day for exercise or fit it in when you can, either way make sure you don't allow lethargy to hold you back. Identify with your chosen exercise program and enjoy it.

Postscript

If you have enjoyed reading this presentation half as much as I enjoyed writing it, my work has not been in vain. If you apply these principles in your life, reap the benefits and inspire others to do the same, my joy will be complete. See for yourself how simple it can be to get healthy today with the application of Five Point Plan.

I welcome all feedback and enquiries.

BIBLIOGRAPHY

Books

- Your Bodies: Many Cries For Water, by Dr. Batmanghelidj
- Water & Salt, Your Healers From Within, by Dr. Batmanghelidj
- ABC of asthma, allergies and lupus, by Dr. Batmanghelidj
- Neurotransmitter Histamine, An Alternative Viewpoint, by Dr. Batmanghelidj
- Salt Deficiency, by Martin Lara
- Life Flow One, The Solution For Heart Disease, by Karl Loren
- Uropathy, by Martin Lara
- Amaroli, The Occult Practice of the Ancient Aryans, by John Carmo Rodrigues
- The Golden Fountain, by Coen Van Der Kroon
- Shivambu Gita by Dr. G. K. Thakkar
- Water of Life by John W. Armstrong
- Urotherapy for patients with cancer, by Dr. Joseph Eldor
- Shivambu Kalpa Vidhi by

➤ Healing with whole foods, by Paul Pitchford

➤ Miracle of Fasting, by Paul Bragg

➤ Fasting: A Unique Remedy for A Hundred Ailments, by R.M Metha

➤ Spirulina, The Most Powerful Food On Earth by B.V. Umesh

➤ The Blending Book, by Dr. Ann Wigmore

➤ Juice Diet For Perfect Health, by Dr's Gala

➤ Apple Cider Vinegar – Miracle Health System, by Paul Bragg

➤ Light on Yoga, by BKS Iyengar

➤ Neti, Healing Secrets of Yoga and Ayurveda, by David Frawley

➤ The Healing Power of Mudras, by Rajender Menon

➤ The Five Tibetans, by Christopher S. Kilham

➤ Yoga, Mind and Body, by the Sivananda Yoga Vedanta Centre

➤ Opening The Energy Floodgates Of The Body, by B.K Frantzis

➤ Ancient Secret of the Fountain of Youth: Book 2' (companion to Kelders book)

➤ Sai Baba: The Supreme Doctor, by P. Sivaraman

➤ The Ten Commandments Of Health, by Dr. Jonathan Dao

➤ Bhagavad Gita

➤ Holy Bible

Websites

- www.watercure.com
- www.watercure2.com
- www.shirleys-wellness-café.com
- www.hps-online.com
- www.saisanjeevini.org
- www.spirulina.com
- www.notmilk.com
- www.mercola.com
- www.sproutman.com
- www.healself.org
- www.drbass.com
- www.naturalhygienesociety.org
- www.rawschool.com
- www.whfoods.com
- www.holisticonline.org
- www.vahini.org
- www.sathyasai.org

APPENDICES

Healthy Living Tips

- ➤ Drink the correct amount of pure water each day.
- ➤ Take the correct amount of real salt each day.
- ➤ Compensate with pure water when you drink diuretic drinks.
- ➤ Don't eat, unless you are actually hungry.
- ➤ Eat a primarily alkaline-based diet.
- ➤ Eat raw food regularly.
- ➤ Eat soaked/sprouted seeds.
- ➤ Drink fruit/vegetable juices.
- ➤ Incorporate various exercises into your daily routine.
- ➤ Take time to sit quietly with your eyes closed each day.
- ➤ Breath 'consciously' as much as possible.
- ➤ Take time to visualise yourself as healthy.
- ➤ Drink at least a small amount of your own midstream urine each morning.
- ➤ Chew your food well before swallowing it.
- ➤ Fall asleep each night with a calm mind and pleasant thoughts.

> When you go for a pee, think 'when will I replace the fluid I am losing?'
> Avoid unnatural, artificial and adulterated foods/drinks.
> Make your own colloidal silver and use it both internally and externally.
> Practice fasting regularly.
> Keep your living environment clean and tidy.
> Don't chat on mobile phones.
> Boost essential fatty acid levels with hempseed oil/linseed oil etc.
> Practice the 'inner smile' whenever you think to.
> Before eating a cooked meal, eat a small amount of raw food.
> Sleep on a firm surface.
> Don't eat food late in the evening.
> Combine the food you eat correctly.
> Take spirulina, wheatgrass and other green super foods.
> Eat food slowly and when you are in a calm frame of mind.
> Keep your posture correct as much as possible.
> Stop eating before you get full up.
> Avoid meat and keep dairy products to a minimum.
> When you prepare food, be aware that your thoughts and feelings affect what you are preparing.
> Drink a glass of water half an hour before eating a meal.
> Don't drink too much water for at least an hour after eating (two hours for a big meal).
> Make the most of sunlight on your body.
> Drink the purest water that you can.
> Eat seasonal fruit and vegetables.

➤ Avoid doing anything you need to recover from.

➤ Quit smoking cigarettes.

➤ Don't make decisions based on fear.

➤ Believe in your own body's innate wisdom and self-healing capabilities.

➤ Don't spend too much time around negative people.

➤ Treat yourself to some form of therapy/bodywork from time to time.

➤ Floss your teeth regularly.

➤ Wake up in the morning and sleep at night – avoid shift work.

➤ If you feel hungry but know that it is probably better not to eat, brush your teeth and have a drink of water.

➤ Breathe in a circular fashion whenever you think to.

➤ Avoid eating meat.

➤ Don't lend your energy to negative and defeatist attitudes.

➤ Aim to practice some warm-up exercises/yoga/chi kung/ five tibetans rites for at least five or ten minutes per day.

➤ Know the ingredients of what you eat; always check the labels on packaged foods.

➤ Don't create problems by hurrying and worrying.

➤ Live in the awareness that your body is an infinitely creative self-healing entity.

➤ Avoid tensing muscles that don't need to be tensed.

➤ Take responsibility for your own health and be disciplined when overcoming bad diet and lifestyle habits.

➤ Avoid all cosmetics, toothpastes, shampoos etc that contain a long list of chemicals.

➤ Try to be aware of the many other health hazards in modern life and strive to avoid them or protect yourself against them.

Basic Dietary & Lifestyle Questionnaire

How much water (on it's actual form or in a non-diuretic form, such as herbal tea) do you drink each day?	
What type of water is it? (ie tap, bottled etc)	
How much tea/coffee do you drink each day?	
How much sugar do you put in each cup?	
Do you drink pasteurised milk?	
If so, how much per day?	
What kind of soft drinks do you drink?	
How many per day?	
What type of salt do you use?	
How much salt do you use each day?	
What sort of breakfast do you have?	
What sort of lunch do you have?	
What sort of supper do you have?	
What sort of snacks do you eat between meals?	
Do you eat meat?	
If so, what kind of meat?	

How much meat do you eat per week?	
Do you eat chocolate bars, cakes and biscuits?	
If so, how much per week?	
Do you drink alcohol?	
What kind of alcohol? (include brand names)	
How much per week?	
Do you smoke cigarettes?	
If so, how many per day?	
Do you eat many fresh fruits/vegetables?	
How much per day?	
Is it organic?	
Do you do exercise?	
What sort?	
How much per week?	
Do you ever have constipation/diarrhoea?	
Do you have any mercury/amalgam fillings?	
How many?	
What vaccinations have you had?	
Have you noticed feeling particularly bad, or experiencing any possible side effects from vaccination?	
Have you had any serious illnesses in your life?	
If so, please give details	
Is there any other factors you can think of that may be influencing your health?	

Colloidal Silver

'Colloidal silver is emerging as a miracle of modern medicine'.

- Dr. Harry Magraf

The word 'colloid' can be defined as:

'A system in which finely divided particles, which are approximately 10 to 10,000 angstroms in size, are dispersed within a continuous medium in a manner that prevents them from being filtered easily or settled rapidly.'

Colloidal silver refers to the liquid elixir that is made by electrically suspending colloids of pure silver in water, which is the safest and most effective way to absorb silver into the body.

In recent years there has been a growing awareness of the universal benefits of colloidal silver, with the emergence of many small companies selling it through websites and small adverts. Colloidal silver is widely acknowledged as an agent for killing bacteria, viruses and fungi, whilst raising the effectiveness of the immune system and purging the body of accumulated toxins. As with other precious metals such as gold and platinum, silver has a unique place in holistic healing and can dramatically improve the lives of those who utilize it correctly, primarily by drinking small amounts of silver colloid in pure water.

It is used to be common practice to put a silver coin in a bottle of milk to keep it from souring, or in a bottle of water to purify it. The ancient Greeks and the Romans used to put silver into their urns to keep the water fresh and in the middle age royalty eating with silver utensils were not affected so badly by the Great Plague. In 1938 a patent was placed on colloidal silver and production was drastically reduced in favour of the new breed of antibiotics that were hitting the market. Today we are aware of the limitations and dangers of such antibiotics, setting the stage nicely for the re-emergence of silver as the natural antibiotic alternative of choice. The restrictions placed on colloidal silver in 1938 have since been removed and anyone can now make colloidal silver from home, using simply an electrical supply source (a 9 volt battery will suffice), 2 pure silver rods and some crocodile clips.

A very large number of diseases can be helped or cured with the aid of colloidal silver, so many in fact, that if the knowledge was widely available to the population the sales of pharmaceutical alternatives would take a nose dive.

A regular antibiotic prescribed by doctor may kill around 6 harmful parasites or bacteria, which is why choosing the correct the type is very important. Colloidal silver, on the other hand, killed around 650 harmful parasites and bacteria within 6 minutes (as reported by Jim Powell in the Science Digest, 1978). Not only is colloidal silver far more universal, it is also completely free from the damaging side effects of modern antibiotics, it is so non-toxic that it can safely be used as an eye drop for babies.

Some of the most popular uses for colloidal silver are for

repairing a weakened immune system and overcoming parasitic and bacterial infections, such as food poisoning. Other uses include eczema, arthritis and even multiple sclerosis and cancer to name just a few.

A CLOSER LOOK AT COLLOIDAL SILVER

'Thanks to our eye opening research, silver is emerging as a wonder of modern medicine. An antibiotic kills perhaps half a dozen different disease organisms, but silver kills some 650.'

- Jim Powell, Science Digest, 1978

The colloidal silver has been used to successfully treat the following complaints:

- ➤ Acne
- ➤ AIDS
- ➤ Allergies
- ➤ Appendicitis
- ➤ Athlete's Foot
- ➤ Bladder infection
- ➤ Blood parasites
- ➤ Blood poisoning
- ➤ Boils
- ➤ Bubonic Plague
- ➤ Burns
- ➤ Cancers
- ➤ Candida
- ➤ Chilblains
- ➤ Cholera

- ➢ Colitis
- ➢ Conjunctivitis
- ➢ Cystitis
- ➢ Dandruff
- ➢ Dermatitis
- ➢ Diabetes
- ➢ Dysentery
- ➢ Eczema
- ➢ Encephalitis
- ➢ Fibrositis
- ➢ Gastritis
- ➢ Gonorrhea
- ➢ Hay Fever
- ➢ Herpes
- ➢ Food poisoning
- ➢ Indigestion
- ➢ Jaundice
- ➢ Leprosy
- ➢ Leukemia
- ➢ Lupus
- ➢ Lyme Disease
- ➢ Keratitis
- ➢ Malaria
- ➢ Meningitis
- ➢ Neurasthenia
- ➢ Parasitic infections

- Pleurisy
- Pneumonia
- Prostate
- Pain
- Psoriasis
- Purulent Ophthalmia
- Rhinitis
- Ringworm
- Scarlet Fever
- Seborrhea
- Septic conditions of the eyes, ears, mouth and throat
- Septicemia
- Shingles
- Skin cancer
- Staph. infections
- Stomach flu
- Strep. infections
- Syphilis
- Thrush, yeast infection
- Thyroid
- Tonsillitis
- Toxema
- Tuberculosis
- Ulcerated stomach virus, all forms
- Warts
- Whooping Cough
- Yeast infections

BENEFITS OF COLLOIDAL SILVER

- ➢ Iron clad immune system
- ➢ More energy
- ➢ Shining eyes
- ➢ Purging accumulated toxins
- ➢ Invigorating electrical stimulation of body
- ➢ Anti-aging
- ➢ Counters parasitic and bacterial infection

FACTS

- ➢ Flower cuttings often live for twice as long, when kept in a cup of water containing colloidal silver.
- ➢ Silver wires can be placed into a hot bathtub and connected to a battery for a while to make a colloidal silver bath.
- ➢ Since ancient times, silver has been closely associated with the moon and lunar influences as well as the goddess Isis and all things flexible, creative, and emotionally intelligent.
- ➢ Based on evidence found on islands in the Aegean Sea, mankind has practiced the science of separating silver from lead at least as far back as 3000 BC.
- ➢ Other precious metals can be electrically colloided into water. Gold is known for its mood-enhancing qualities and copper has rejuvenating effect on the joints, skin and hair.

MAKING COLLOIDAL SILVER

- ➢ It's easy to make colloidal silver, all that is needed is:
- ➢ 2 small crocodile clips,
- ➢ 3, 9 volt battery terminals
- ➢ 3, 9 volt batteries

> ➢ 2 short lengths of 99.9% pure silver wire.
> ➢ A glass of suitable water
> ➢ Small cleaning pad and cloth

Fill a glass with warm water, connect the batteries to the silver wires, put the silver wires into the crocodile clips and place them into the water as parallel as possible and about an inch or two apart. From the positive wire you will soon see whispy clouds of silver

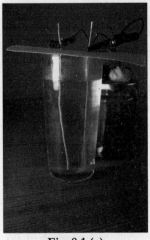

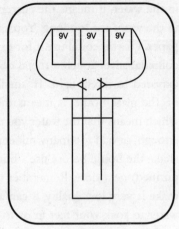

Fig. 8.1 (a)   **Fig. 8.1 (b)**

Fig. 8.1 (a) Home made colloidal silver using hot filtered water shows the cloudy 'tyndall effect' that the tiny silver particles make when being electrically released into the liquid. The three batteries are resting on a jar of molasses.

Fig. 8.1 (b) Diagram of the scientific set-up (3 batteries, glass, crocodile clips etc).

disperse into the water. When the water looks cloudy, the colloidal silver is ready. Give it a stir and put it into a dark, glass bottle with a plastic cap. You've now got a very beneficial and safe medicine that can benefit millions around the world for the price of water.

There are more sophisticated methods of making colloidal silver, but this one works well. Avoid mineral water or straight tap water. Distilled water gives higher quality colloidal silver. Putting a few tiny grains of salt in the cup (to give it more conductivity) will make the process of making colloidal silver quicker and using hot water (approximately 90 degrees), the process of making a pint only takes a few minutes.

After the colloidal silver is made, one of the silver wires should be a grey/dark silver in colour. Use a non-metallic kitchen pad and cloth to clean it before the next use. If small flakes of black appear in the water, it means the current is too high or the rods have been in the water for too long. You can still use it if you have some filter paper. Or you could use it for external use. Remember not to let the colloidal silver touch a metal object (such as a metal spoon) or get exposed to direct light. If small silver particles fall to the bottom of the glass bottle, it means the electrical suspension is dropping which means that the water you used probably was not quite purified enough, or had too many minerals in it. It is still worth keeping, just shake the bottle before use - but try to use better water (distilled or purified) next time. Remember that, even if the colloidal silver you make is very low quality, it can always be used in a bucket with hot water to soak your feet in or to use on the skin. In emergencies, it is always better to have some low quality colloidal silver than no colloidal silver at all.

As the battery loses power, the colloidal silver will lower in quality and take longer to make. If possible, use a rechargeable 9-volt battery and re-charge it after it has been used a few times.

1. Fill a clean glass container with suitable water*.

2. Add a very tiny amount of sea/rock salt or baking soda if necessary**.

3. Place the two silver wires over a glass container using the plastic holder provided in this kit (or by putting two holes in

the top of the lid of your container).

4. Clip the two crocodile clips to the ends of the wires.

5. Connect the 3, 9-volt batteries.

6. Wait for a suitable length of time***.

7. Remove the wires and disconnect the batteries.

8. Stir with a clean, plastic spoon.

9. Pour into a dark glass bottle.

10. Clean the silver wires with both the souring pad and the cloth.

*Suitable water

The distilled, de-ionised or reverse osmosis water will produce the highest quality solution. The distilled water is completely 'empty', ie – contains 0 ppm impurity whereas the de-ionised/ the reverse osmosis water contains about 1 ppm. There's very little difference between them. Because there will be less electrolyte in these waters as compared with, say filtered tap water, the time it takes to make a suitably strong colloidal silver preparation will be longer.

**Adding electrolyte

Adding a very tiny amount of real sea/rock salt or baking soda will speed up the process, as will heating the water (which I do by placing the glass jar in a large saucepan with boiled hot water in it). Literally, put just about the tiniest amount of salt/baking soda that you can. Put too much electrolyte in the water and the silver particles are likely to fall out of suspension and rest at the bottom of the bottle.

***Timing

Generally speaking, using 3 fresh 9-volt batteries and a 500ml glass container with distilled water at room temperature, it should take about 25 minutes to create a 5ppm colloidal silver solution. Heating the water and adding electrolyte can speed up the process significantly. Experiment for yourself, you'll know when the solution is ready because one of the silver wires will have a grey/black coating on it. If you are using pure distilled/de-ionised/reverse osmosis water with no electrolyte, you will not see any wispy clouds of silver 'smoke' coming from the silver wire (this is known as the Tyndall effect) and will only know that the solution is indeed colloidal silver by taste and by seeing the residue left on the wire or by using an electronic PPM testing device.

In an emergency, say if you burn yourself, you can run the hot tap until it is as hot as it gets, fill a pint glass and put the silver wires in it. You're crude silver preparation will only take a minute. This kind of preparation can be used for plants, topical applications and general household hygiene purposes.

NB:

> Keep the silver preparation away from direct light and strong electro-magnetic fields (such as near hi-fi speakers).

> If any dust gets into the preparation as you are making it, filter it using a funnel and un-bleached brown coffee filter paper.

> Remember that the batteries will lose power each time you make a batch of silver solution. Researchers have found about 30 volts to be ideal. 3 fully charged 9-volt batteries gives 27 volts. Use a battery re-charger if you plan to make colloidal silver/silver solution regularly.

A wide range of higher quality colloidal silver generators is available primarily via the Internet and mail order companies. Below are some examples of different types of commercially sold generators.

So simple it's beautiful. The ultimate lightweight colloidal silver generator makes use of a special microchip current converter. Costs

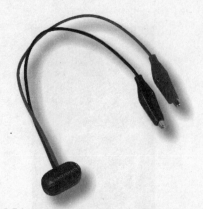

Fig. 8.2 Light weight colloidal silver generator

about £40 and is available from various Internet websites.

A simple home colloidal silver generator can be bought on the Internet for about £25-60 or made for about £10-15.

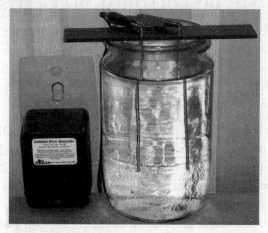

Fig. 8.3 Simple home colloidal silver generator

Commercial colloidal silver generators, such as the one pictured above can produce over five gallons of high quality colloidal silver per hour.

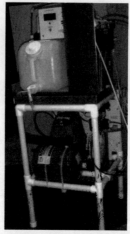

Fig. 8.4 Commercial colloidal silver generator

WHY I MAKE AND PROMOTE SIMPLE, EASY-TO-DUPLICATE, DIY COLLOIDAL SILVER KITS

In 1999 I was told about how effective colloidal silver was and decided straight away to buy a kit and start making it myself; for myself and anyone else I knew who wanted to try some. Since then I've been making it regularly and have distributed probably well over two thousand bottles and kits in India and the UK.

As well as supplying local shops with bottles and DIY kits, I tell many people I meet about how easy it is to make and what an excellent opportunity it is to help other people overcome illness and raise immunity. I become ever more enthusiastic about colloidal silver every time I get positive feedback and it never ceases to amaze me, how such a simple preparation can help cure such a wide range of illnesses. I believe if every household should have a colloidal silver generator; the world would be a much better place to live.

If you have benefited from colloidal silver, I urge you to make colloidal silver for friends/family/pets/plants and, if you have the time, buy the various components in this kit, duplicate it and teach others how to make colloidal silver. For people who are health conscious and like to help others, it is very rewarding work.

Colloidal silver is not 'just another natural health supplement', it has the all-round goodness to revolutionise the worlds health.

This is how I got started with colloidal silver:

> Experimented with making and taking colloidal silver.

> Noticed the benefits.

> Made a few extra bottles.

> Offered it friends/family who were receptive to the idea (always give a photocopied/printed A4 leaflet for them to read).

> Collected some testimonials.

> Duplicated the kit and taught other people how to make and distribute it (always give photocopied/printed instructions and general information).

TESTIMONIES

Below are some testimonies from my experiences with friends and acquaintances over the last few years:

'My fingers tips and eyes were yellow as I had been suffering from jaundice for many months. After taking 20ml of colloidal silver every day for 5 days, all the symptoms disappeared and now I feel better than ever. I was very happy and surprised'.

- Vishnu, Goa

'I had conjunctivitis in my right eye for over 2 months and after 3 washes with colloidal silver it went away completely, I was so impressed that I bought a kit and started making it for myself'.

- Mike, London

'Chemotherapy, surgery, antibiotics and radiation had not got rid of the lumps under my breast. Then I was given a supply of Colloidal Silver and a sheet containing simple dietary advice so I started taking it. Within 2 days I felt better in myself and within 7 weeks the lumps had completely disappeared. It's now been 6 months, I feel great and people are telling me I look 10 years younger! Just so you know, I told my doctor that his advice wasn't as good as the Colloidal Silver and he got angry, saying 'don't talk to me like that!'. I walked out of his office, saying 'It's not about you, it's about me!'. The whole episode had been a learning process and I'm very grateful I discovered Colloidal Silver when I did otherwise, I may well be dead now'.

- Jan, Portsmouth

'Travelling around Asia for so long was starting to make me ill, my gums were bleeding whenever I brushed my teeth and I felt tired most of the time. I started taking about 50ml of Colloidal Silver in sips through the day and seemed to feel better within a few hours. The gums cleared up in 2 days'.

- David, Ireland

'I never forget to take my morning swig of colloidal silver, it seems to give me a very nice energy boost and I'm noticing my eyes are getting brighter'.

- Iris, Bournemouth

'I had this horrible shingles around my chest and stomach - nothing seemed to be working. Someone recommended trying colloidal silver so I did, twice a day. Amazingly, the condition showed signs of improvement after only a few days and after a week I felt completely fine again'.

- Tony, London

'For Years now I've been making colloidal silver in my organic 'Earthfoods' store in Bournemouth, Dorset, I must admit in the past I have only used it for prevention, it must have been working very well, because I never really caught anything, that is until I got to Kathmandu Nepal, where I caught the 'Kathmandu Quick Step', however at that time I was industrious in making it for myself with a simple generator, showing the tourists, a Dutch medical team, the Hoteliers and a Canadian Nurse. All of these people (over 20) had never heard of it, and at least 75%were suffering from Delhi Belly! Well, you can guess the rest - a few big swigs for 3 or 4 days and yes, everybody was cured! So the amazing quickness of the CS surprised everyone at the Hotel.

I usually use de-ionized water, that time I used the bottled water you can buy there (just make sure the top seal is not broken), they were all instantly converted and no doubt they too will now spread the news about the wonderful healing properties of CS, at virtually no expense, just a few pounds outlay.'

-Carl, Bournemouth

'Whilst filling up the charcoal water filter, I accidentally poured five litres of boiling water all down my left shin. It was horrific, my skin was bubbling and seriously burned. I didn't go to the hospital as advised but rather made up a large batch of low quality colloidal silver (in a bucket of hot water) and poured it all over my shin regularly.

I also applied urine to my shin. Many people were worried for me and a nurse said I was crazy because it could get seriously infected. When that same nurse passed by my house two weeks later she said she had never seen anything like it before. My shin was 95% better. Now there is no sign at all that it had been so badly burned.'

- James, Bournemouth

'4 children got a stomach bug on farm where travelling people live. I think it may have been because of dog pooh lying around. Their symptoms were diarrhoea, vomiting and a slight fever - maybe due to the dog pooh. A few cupfuls of colloidal silver every few hours, and all the children were fine in 6-12 hours...

'A tooth pain suddenly came in a root canal. Since rinsing my mouth with colloidal silver it has been completely pain free...'

'A friend did too much cocaine nasally and has a sinus problem since. She says the sniffing of colloidal silver helped her.'

- Crispin, Bournemouth

'I had Venereal disease for over two years and after about two months of taking colloidal silver every morning, it is completely gone'.

- Martin, London

'I started making my own colloidal silver in October 2007 and since then have noticed a significant difference in several aspects of my life. The first (and most noticeable) effect was when I had an abscess on a tooth and did not have access to a dentist. I decided to swill colloidal silver around my mouth at regular intervals and after only about 45 minutes the pain had stopped. By the next day everything had cleared up and there was no need to visit a dentist.

Other results have been recurrent mouth ulcers being immediately cleared up from gargling and it has completely turned around the health of my teenage daughter's health. Before colloidal silver she suffered from IBS and now I would say it is 90% better, she's fourteen years old and loves to make her own colloidal silver in the kitchen and always takes a bottle with her when she goes away.'

Lorna, Bournemouth

COLLOIDAL SILVER AND ANIMALS

I have also had successes using colloidal silver with animals. Lizzy is a beach dog in Goa and was the runt of the litter. In her first year of life, she developed a nasty lung condition that had already killed a few other dogs that week. One afternoon, I found a small group of tourists gathering around Lizzy, who by this point seemed to be nearly dead. I watched as everyone fussed and worried about the poor dog and then suddenly had an idea. "Hey, I'll get some colloidal silver and we can squirt it into her mouth…wait there!" I said as I dashed home to get a bottle and pipette. I soon returned and began squirting colloidal silver under the dogs tongue every minute or so. The result was so quick that I'm sure onlookers weren't sure what to think. Within about ten minutes Lizzy's eyes had opened, she was walking around and had recovered her appetite to eat the chicken soup we had previously made for her! I poured a little colloidal silver on all the food we gave to her over the next couple of days and she made a 100% recovery. In fact she seemed stronger and more vibrant than before she got sick - another triumph for home made colloidal silver!

Once I helped a cow with a nasty open wound on its foot get better by pouring a crude colloidal silver solution on to it every day. I've also had reports of how it helps dogs with worms in their guts and how once it restored the health of a famous Danish race horse that the vets had virtually given up on. So if you are producing colloidal silver for yourself, I suggest making a bit for any sick animal you might know about. It can't do any harm and it may just restore it's life back into a healthy one.

Q & A

How much should I take?

A general recommendation is about 10 ml every day as maintenance and 10ml regularly throughout the day to beat the illnesses. Suggested doses vary according to the strength of the solution amongst other factors. Some people are taking much more than these recommendations and are suffering no adverse effects at all. As with all natural remedies, follow your instincts and if it feels right to take more, then go ahead. If you find that you are extremely sick with food poisoning, you may want to take a small sip as often as possible for a while.

How should I take it?

Try to space it out through the day but there's no fixed guidelines as such. Do not use a metal spoon as it ruins the electrical charge of the colloidal silver. It's also worthwhile to swill it around your mouth and gargle with it before swallowing to kill the germs in and around the mouth as well.

What other uses are there?

Rub on cuts, into infected ears and gums, spray onto food, mix with suspect water, clean utensils with it, rub into scalp, give to poorly animals or mix with water and give to plants. Be creative, as no doubt the full potential of colloidal silver has not been realised yet.

Can I take too much?

Yes, but people don't suffer long-term side effects, even if they exceed the recommended doses by many times. The body can only process so much at a time, so if you are taking too much, the body will expel the unused silver through the urine and pores in the skin. It would be a good idea to take something like yoghurt/curd to re-build the friendly intestinal flora that may be slightly diminished at the higher doses. A small amount every day is usually all that is needed.

I read on the Internet that it was dangerous to ingest heavy metals and that your skin will go grey if you do. Is this true?

The condition they are referring to is Argyria, which is a cosmetic condition that leaves the skin on the face looking slightly silvery. It is thought to be due to selenium and Vitamin E deficiency in combination with very high levels of silver in the blood stream. You would have to be drinking many litres each month for a long time to develop this condition, so in truth, the only people who should be concerned are researchers who are currently drinking massive amounts of Colloidal Silver each day and are deficient in Selenium and Vitamin E. The cases of Argyria are being touted by the pharmaceutical complex are yet another tactic designed to discourage people from finding out about just how safe, cheap and thoroughly effective modern-day colloidal silver is.

AN UPDATE ON COLLOIDAL SILVER AND DISINFORMATION, JULY 2008-07-20

Most of my core research into colloidal silver was done from around 2000-2005, so I hadn't entered the keywords 'colloidal silver' into the google.com search engine for some time. When I did last week I was appalled at what I found. It seems that certain 'powers that be' have seriously clamped down on honest information regarding colloidal silver and replaced it with half-truth and downright lies.

Certain readers may find it hard to believe that some kind of a clandestine / semi-clandestine group would spend so much time and money suppressing something like colloidal silver, however in my experience this is exactly what happens when something genuinely revolutionary begins to surface in the public consciousness.

The US passed a law, a few years ago that prohibited a website from both providing information about the health benefits of colloidal silver and selling the kits to make it. I remember that this meant many small businesses were harassed and put out of business by the FDA. Things seem to have got worse since then.

I'll say this as straight as I can; there are snakes out there on the Internet and TV whose job it is to hoodwink, bamboozle and lead you astray. With multi-billion dollar empires to protect and virtually unlimited funds to protect these empires by any means necessary, disinformation has become a highly profitable business.

'They' will tell you that your skin will turn silver if you take colloidal silver, or you'll die from heavy metal poisoning, yet 'they' are not who they seem. 'They', in my opinion, are professional 'bought and paid for' disinformation artists. Sure, if you drink litres of crude colloidal silver each day you may develop a cosmetic skin condition but this kind of intake is totally unnecessary as a small sip is enough. Beware of websites that may come across as 'oh so authoritative' or 'oh so professional' yet whose primary aim is to cause fear and turn you off colloidal silver.

I first came across this appalling website a few years ago. At the time I was promoting and distributing colloidal silver bottles and generators. On occasion, someone would say negative things about me and the colloidal silver, which left me confused and slightly upset. I wondered 'where on earth are these folk getting their ideas from?' It is one thing to be sceptical; it is another to instigate an argument by presenting clearly false information dressed up as fact. So I went online and typed 'colloidal silver' into the search engine in order to find what the 'anti colloidal silver' contingent was saying. What I found, right up near the top of the list on page one (since then quackwatch is now at the very top, every time) was a link to Barratt's site. The entry headline read 'Colloidal silver: Risk without benefit…' I clicked on the link and made my way to the colloidal silver section. What I read made me realise quite quickly that this character Steven Barrett must surely be on a pay-off from some shadowy group or other. So I clicked on other sections on the website and realised that he is discrediting all manner of other natural healthcare remedies and systems from Acupuncture to WaterCure, using sensational spin and downright misinformation.

Occasionally, there are people who say the product is dangerous and that I should not be distributing it. I thought about my detractors, who seemed so sure that colloidal silver was a menace to society and tried to sympathise with them. I guess if someone wants to have a quick browse around the topic of colloidal silver on the Internet and then chance upon a site like quackwatch.com, they can be forgiven for believing the lies perpetrated by the anti-colloidal silver/anti-natural healthcare circus. Even without clicking on the quackwatch.com link, a very casual browser could be dissuaded from ever trying colloidal silver by simply reading the three words 'risk without benefit'. I met someone who said to me once 'I went on the net and saw that colloidal silver is dangerous'. Upon further questioning, this person had actually not even opened any website at all, other than the google.com search engine. The first link they came across was quackwatch.com and the headline was enough for them not to even bother opening the link. 'I suspected it was all snake oil all along and the website confirmed it'. Three words – risk without benefit – that's all it can take to deter someone from the amazing colloidal silver.

At the end of the day, I have sympathy for these misled people. They'll no doubt run to the doctor for antibiotics when they get sick and that is their free will choice. I have less sympathy for the rascal Steven Barrett and his god-forsaken parrots, incessantly proclaiming the dangers and ineffectiveness of 'alternative' healthcare. The knock-on effect of deliberately mis-informing the public about important healthcare issues can lead to untold suffering and unnecessarily premature deaths.

Summary

The weakened immune systems and parasitic/bacterial 'infections' are the cause of suffering and death for millions of people around the world. Colloidal silver is virtually free to make, safe to use and highly effective against hundreds of illnesses. It simultaneously raises the immune system whilst purging the body of accumulated toxins and killing harmful parasites and bacteria. This makes it a life-saving preparation of extremely high value to our society.

Shivambu Kalpa Vidhi – Damar Tantra

The Shivambu Kalpa Vidhi is a part of the five-thousand year old text titled, Damar Tantra.

Verses 1-21

> Oh Parvati! I shall expound to you the recommended actions and rituals of Shivambu Kalpa that confers numerous benefits. Those well versed in the scriptures have carefully specified certain vessels for the purpose. (1)

> Utensils made from the following materials are recommended: Gold, Silver, Copper, Bronze, Brass, Iron, Clay, Ivory, Glass, Wood from sacred trees, Bones, Leather and Leaves. (2, 3)

> The Shivambu (one's own urine) should be collected in a utensil made of any of these materials. Among them, clay utensils are better, copper are by far the best. (4)

> The intending practitioner of the therapy should abjure salty or bitter foods, should not over-exert himself, should take a light meal in the evening, should sleep on the ground, and should control and master his senses. (5)

> The sagacious practitioner should get up when three

> quarters of the night have elapsed, and should pass urine while facing the east. (6)

> ➤ The wise one should leave out the first and the last portions of the urine, and collect only the middle portion. This is considered the best procedure. (7)

> ➤ Just as there is poison in the mouth and the tail of the serpent, O Parvati, it is even so in the case of the flow of Shivambu. (8)

> ➤ Shivambu (urine) is heavenly nectar, which is capable of destroying senility and diseases. The practitioner of Yoga should take it before proceeding with his other rituals. (9)

> ➤ After cleansing the mouth, and performing the other essential morning functions, one should drink one's own clear urine, which is the annihilator of senility and diseases. (10)

> ➤ One who drinks Shivambu for one month will be purified internally. Drinking it for two months stimulates and energizes the senses. (11)

> ➤ Drinking it for three months destroys all diseases and frees one from all troubles. By drinking it for five months, one acquires divine vision and freedom from all diseases. (12)

> ➤ Continuation of the practice for six months makes the practitioner highly intelligent and proficient in the scriptures, and if the duration extends to seven months, the practitioner acquires extraordinary strength. (13)

> ➤ If the practice is continued for eight months, one acquires a permanent glow like that of gold, and if it is continued for nine months, one is freed from tuberculosis and leprosy. (14)

> ➤ Ten months of this practice makes one a veritable treasury of luster. Eleven months of it would purify all the organs of the body. (15)

- ➢ A man who has continued the practice for a year becomes the equal of the sun in radiance. He who has continued for two years conquers the element of Earth. (16)

- ➢ If the practice is continued for three years, one conquers the element of Water, and if it is continued for four years, the element Light is also conquered. (17)

- ➢ He, who continues the practice for five years conquers the element Air, and he who continues it for seven years conquers pride. (18)

- ➢ Continuation of the practice for eight years enables one to conquer all the important elements of Nature, and continuation of it for nine years frees one from the cycle of birth and death. (19)

- ➢ One who has continued the practice for ten years can fly through the air without effort. One who has continued it for eleven years is able to hear the voice of his soul (inner self). (20)

- ➢ He who has continued the practice for twelve years will live so long as the moon and the stars last. He is not troubled by dangerous animals such as snakes, and no poisons can kill him. He cannot be consumed by fire, and can float on water just like wood. (21)

Comparing non-toxic foods chart

NON-TOXIC FOODS	Toxicity	Raw Edibility	Taste Appeal	Digestive Ease	Digest Efficiency	Protein Adequacy	Vitamin Adequacy	Mineral Salt Adequacy	Essential Fatty Acids	Fuel Value	
ITEM:	100~0	0~10	0~10	0~10	0~6	0~5	0~5	0~5	0~5	0~40	Total:
Apple	0	10	10	10	10	3	5	4	3	40	95
Apricot	0	10	10	10	10	5	5	5	3	40	98
Avocado	0	10	8	8	7	5	5	5	5	40	93
Banana	0	10	10	10	10	5	5	5	5	40	100
Berries	0	10	8	10	10	5	5	5	5	35	93
Cantaloupe	0	10	10	10	10	5	5	5	3	40	98
Cherimoya	0	10	10	10	10	5	4	5	4	40	98
Cherry	0	10	10	10	10	5	5	5	4	40	99
Corn	0	10	5	9	9	5	5	5	5	40	93
Cucumber	0	10	5	6	6	5	5	5	3	5	50
Date	0	10	10	10	10	4	3	5	3	40	95

Fig	0	10	10	10	10	5	4	5	5	40	99
Grapefruit	0	10	9	10	10	3	5	4	2	25	78
Grapes	0	10	10	10	10	5	4	4	4	40	97
Mango	0	10	10	10	10	4	5	3	5	40	97
Orange	0	10	10	10	10	5	5	5	2	40	97
Papaya	0	10	10	10	10	4	5	4	2	40	95
Peas	0	10	7	7	9	4	5	5	4	40	91
Peach	0	10	10	10	10	4	5	4	2	40	95
Pear	0	10	10	10	10	3	4	3	4	40	94
Pecan	0	10	7	7	5	5	3	5	5	40	87
Pineapple	0	10	10	10	10	2	4	3	4	40	93
Plum	0	10	10	10	10	3	4	3	3	35	88
Potato, sweet	0	5	4	4	5	5	5	5	5	40	78
Sesame seeds	0	8	4	6	4	5	3	5	5	40	80
Sprouts	0	9	5	8	8	5	5	5	5	0	50
Strawberry	0	10	10	10	10	4	5	4	5	30	88
Sunflower seeds	0	8	5	7	7	5	3	5	5	40	85
Tangerine	0	10	10	10	10	3	5	4	2	40	94
Tomato	0	10	10	10	10	5	5	5	4	20	79
Watermelon	0	10	10	10	10	4	5	4	4	40	97

The postural theory of hypochondria

I added this to the appendices because I am noticing many of my friends and associates sitting for long hours each day at a PC with a terrible posture. As the computer revolution continues, the problems associated with bad posture will also continue.

The word hypochondria is derived from the ancient Greek terms 'hypo', which means below, and 'chondros', which means cartilage, and it refers to a set of symptoms which were thought to have been caused by a disorder of the anatomical organs beneath the cartilages of the ribs. This included disorders of the liver and spleen, but there is also some indication that it referred to a disorder originating beneath the cartilage tip at the base of the breastbone. This area includes the base of the heart, and the junction of the food pipe and the stomach. It is crossed by the diaphragm, which is the main muscle responsible for breathing. The solar plexus, which supplies nerves to every part of the chest and abdomen, is also below the tip of the breastbone.

The symptoms of hypochondria include:

➢ Backache

> Neck ache

> Upper abdominal pain

> Palpitations

> Breathlessness

> Faintness

> Fatigue

> Pain in the lower left and right side of the chest

> Kidney pain

> A variety of others which all have undetectable causes

The cause of hypochondria had remained a mystery until the publication of an essay entitled 'The Matter Of Framework' in 1980. This essay proposed that poor posture strained the spine and compressed the chest and abdomen to cause a multitude of varied and alternating symptoms.

This concept was devised between 1975 and 1979 and has since been referred to as 'The Posture Theory' The theory was improved between 1994 and 1999 to show that ailment is more common in people who have a stooped spinal deformity and who also have a flat chest.

This is because the combination of those features results in the torso buckling when the person slouches forward, and in this movement the midriff acts as a hinge. Consequently, the midriff moves backwards, and the chest rotates forwards and downwards, toward the abdomen, which rotates forwards and upwards.

This produces mechanical forces along that axis which directly compresses the:

> Lower chest

> Diaphragm

> Stomach
> Liver
> Spleen

and secondarily compresses the:

> Heart
> Lungs
> Colon
> Kidneys

and drives the lower tip of the breastbone inward towards the solar plexus.

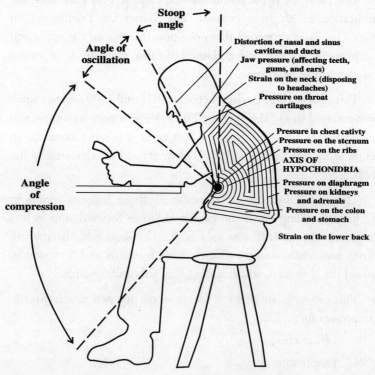

Stoop angle →

← Angle of oscillation

Angle of compression

Distortion of nasal and sinus cavities and ducts
Jaw pressure (affecting teeth, gums, and ears)
Strain on the neck (disposing to headaches)
Pressure on throat cartilages

Pressure in chest cativty
Pressure on the sternum
Pressure on the ribs
AXIS OF HYPOCHONIDRIA
Pressure on diaphragm
Pressure on kidneys and adrenals
Pressure on the colon and stomach

Strain on the lower back

Bhagavad Gita, Chapter 6 - The Yoga of Meditation

'One must elevate, not degrade, oneself

By one's own mind.

The mind alone is one's friend

As well as one's enemy.

The mind is the friend

Of those who have control over it,

And the mind acts like an enemy

For those who do not control it.

One who has control over the mind

Is tranquil in heat and cold,

In pleasure and pain, and in honor and dishonor;

And is ever steadfast with the Supreme Self.

A yogi is called Self-realized

Who is satisfied with knowledge

And understanding of the Self,

Who is equanimous, who has control over the senses,

And to whom a cloud, a stone, and gold are the same.

A person is considered superior

Who is impartial towards companions,

Friends, enemies, neutrals, arbiters,

Haters, relatives, saints, and sinners.

Let the yogi seated in solitude and alone

Having mind and senses under control

And free from desires and attachments for possessions,

Try constantly to contemplate on the Supreme Self.

The yogi should sit on a firm seat

That is neither too high nor too low,

Covered with sacred Kusha grass,

A deerskin, and a cloth,

One over the other, in a clean spot.

Sitting and concentrating the mind

On a single object,

Controlling the thoughts

And the activities of the senses,

Let the yogi practice meditation for self-purification.

Hold the waist, spine, chest, neck, and head erect,

Motionless and steady, fix the eyes and the mind

Steadily between the eye brows,

And do not look around.

With serene and fearless mind;

Practicing celibacy; having the mind under control

And thinking of Me; let the yogi sit

And have Me as the supreme goal.

Thus, by always keeping the mind fixed on the Self,

The yogi whose mind is subdued attains peace

Of the Supreme nirvana by uniting with Me.

This yoga is not possible, O Arjuna,

For the one who eats too much,

Or who does not eat at all;

Who sleeps too much,

Or who keeps awake.

But, for the one who is moderate

In eating, recreation, working,

Sleeping, and waking,

This yoga destroys sorrow.

A person is said to have achieved yoga,

The union with the Self,

When the perfectly disciplined mind

Gets freedom from all desires,

And becomes absorbed in the Self alone.'

Poignant Quotes

NATURAL HEALTHCARE

'He who is of calm and happy nature will hardly feel the pressure of age, but to him who is of an opposite disposition youth and age are equally a burden.'

- Plato

'Though I have had two serious illnesses in my life, I believe that man has little need to drug himself. 999 cases out of a thousand can be brought round by means of a well-regulated diet, water and earth treatment and similar household remedies.'

- Gandhi

'Everything in excess is opposed to nature.'

- Hippocrates

'Misdirected life force is the activity in disease process. Disease has no energy save what it borrows from the life of the organism. It is by adjusting the life force that healing must be brought about, *and it is the sun as transformer and distributor of primal spiritual energy that must be utilized in this process, for life and the sun are so intimately connected.'*

- Buddha

'Look deep into nature, and then you will understand everything better.'

- Albert Einstein

'Would you believe that perfect, sickness-free health is natural and normal? That disease and suffering are abnormal, unnatural and unnecessary?'

- T C Fry

ALLOPATHIC MEDICINE

'The medical monopoly or medical trust, euphemistically called the American Medical Association, is not merely the meanest monopoly ever organized, but the most arrogant, dangerous and despotic organisation which ever managed a free people in this or any other age. Any and all methods of healing the sick by means of safe, simple and natural remedies are sure to be assailed and denounced by the arrogant leaders of the AMA doctors' trust as fakes, frauds and humbugs.'

-J.W Hodge, M.D

'They certainly give very strange names to diseases.'

- Plato

'If there is evidence that HIV causes AIDS, there should

be scientific documents which either singly or collectively demonstrate that fact, at least with a high probability. There is no such document.'

- Dr. Kary Mullis, Biochemist,
1993 Nobel Prize for Chemistry.

SPIRITUAL GUIDANCE

'Love and serve all humanity.

Assist everyone.

Be happy, be courteous.

Be a dynamo of irrepressible joy.

Recognize God and goodness in every face.

There is no saint without a past and no sinner without a future.

Praise everyone. If you cannot praise someone, let them out of your life.

Be original, be inventive.

Be courageous. Take courage again and again.

Do not imitate; be strong, be upright.

Do not lean on the crutches of others.

Think with your own head. Be yourself.

All perfection and every divine virtue are hidden within you. Reveal them to the world.

Wisdom, too, is already within you. Let it shine forth.

Let the Lord's grace set you free.

Let your life be that of the rose; in silence, it speaks the language of fragrance.'

- Herakhan Babaji

'Begin challenging your own assumptions. Your assumptions are your windows to the world. Scrub them off every once in while, or the light won't come in.'

- Alan Alda

'This New Life is endless, and even after my physical death it will be kept alive by those who live the life of complete renunciation of falsehood, lies, hatred, anger, greed and lust; and who, to accomplish all this, do no lustful actions, do no harm to anyone, do no backbiting, do not seek material possessions or power, who accept no homage, neither covet honour nor shun disgrace, and fear no one and nothing; by those who rely wholly and solely on God, and who love God purely for the sake of loving; who believe in the lovers of God and in the reality of Manifestation, and yet do not expect any spiritual or material reward; who do not let go the hand of Truth, and who, without being upset by calamities, bravely and wholeheartedly face all hardships with one hundred percent cheerfulness, and give no importance to caste, creed and religious ceremonies. This New Life will live by itself eternally, even if there is no one to live it.'

- Meher Baba

'Foresight, a good character, and above all a kind heart are the assets required for a peaceful life.'

- Shirdi Sai Baba

'Sitting quietly, doing nothing, spring comes, and the grass grows by itself.'

- Zen

'The only cure for materialism is the cleansing of the six senses (eyes, ears, nose, tongue, body, and mind). If the senses are clogged, one's perception is stifled. The more it is stifled, the more contaminated the senses become. This creates disorder in the world, and that is the greatest evil of all. Polish the heart, free the six senses and let them function without obstruction, and your entire body and soul will glow.'

-Morehei Ueshiba,
founder of the Aikido martial art